The Medical Practice Performance Management Manual:

How to evaluate employees

Written by:
Courtney Price, Ph.D.
Alys Novak

Published by:
Medical Group Management Association
104 Inverness Terrace East
Englewood, CO 80112
(303) 799-1111

Medical Group Management Association (MGMA) publications are intended to provide current and accurate information and are designed to assist readers in becoming more familiar with the subject matter covered. Such publications are distributed with the understanding that MGMA does not render any legal, accounting or other professional advice that may be construed as specifically applicable to individual situations. No representation or warranties are made concerning the application of legal or other principles discussed by the authors to any specific fact situation, nor is any prediction made concerning how any particular judge, government official or other person who will interpret or apply such principles. Specific factual situations should be discussed with professional advisors.

MGMA
FOUNDED 1926

104 Inverness Terrace East
Englewood, CO 80112

ISBN #1-56829-027-6

Table of contents

Preface

Today there is a definite need to provide a uniform and general framework for performance management that ensures employees know what is expected of them and supervisors know how to establish a job-related basis for planning, managing and evaluating performance. Health care organizations, and especially medical practices, can greatly benefit in improved productivity and cost-effectiveness by using an updated performance management process (PMP).

This book focuses on performance management in the health care setting. It provides medical practice managers with several different performance management measurement tools and introduces various performance management approaches aimed at planning, measuring and improving employee performance. In addition, it will help managers meet national legal requirements for establishing and maintaining a defendable performance management process.

The approaches suggested in the book are designed to meet the needs of medical practices regardless of size and are flexible enough to be tailored to each practice job.

More than performance evaluation forms are included. Tools for the entire performance management process are provided, including a planning worksheet, a mid-year review tool, an evaluation form for both exempt and non-exempt employees, management checklist/guidelines and supervisory tips.

The authors recognize that medical practices can use a variety of different performance management approaches very successfully. There is no one right way, no magical tool. The approaches taken in this text are practical, realistic and designed to fit the realities of both small and large medical practices.

The book incorporates quotes about success stories of health care professionals that demonstrate how effective systems work. In addition, some horror story quotes are included to illustrate the classic problems and pitfalls that can occur because of ineffective performance management.

The book can be used most successfully in conjunction with *The Group Practice Personnel Policies Manual*, which is designed to help medical group practices develop personnel policy manuals and handbooks that reflect not only current societal concerns but also meet the needs of a medical practice. One of the issues this publication deals with briefly is performance management. Since it covers this topic in the context of all the other personnel issues that must be considered, it provides a useful perspective.

The Group Practice Job Description Handbook is another valuable resource. The job description is a powerful tool in ensuring the effectiveness of human resources. This document, if developed and used properly, assists medical practice managers with all their human resource tasks — such as recruitment, performance evaluation and compensation — and thus helps achieve top performance. Since updated job descriptions are the essential foundation for an effective, legally defensible performance management process, the handbook also will serve as a most useful reference.

An ongoing reference for medical practice managers is *Personnel Postscript*. This quarterly newsletter represents

MGMA's commitment to keeping its members informed and updated about human resource practices. Such knowledge will help ensure that group practices are managing their medical employees as productively as possible.

Acknowledgements

This manual is based on the expertise of **Courtney Price** and **Alys Novak**, who served as co-authors.

Acknowledgement also is given to MGMA staff members:

Fred Graham II, Ph.D., FACMGA, senior associate executive director, for spearheading the project; **Dennis L. Barnhardt**, **APR**, director of communications, for managing the production of the manual; **Brenda Hull** for coordinating the project; **Barbara U. Hamilton**, director of the Library Resource Center, and her staff, for gathering reference material for the authors and for reviewing the manual; **Stephanie Wyllyamz**, communications specialist, for desktop publishing and designing the book; and **Deborah V. Kennington**, communications administrative secretary, for proofreading the book.

This manual also has been reviewed for conformity to national legal trends by **Pat Ryan**.

In addition, the manual was reviewed by **Bette A. Waddington**, Management Consulting Service Consultant for MGMA. An expert in health care personnel management who advises members regularly on performance issues, Mrs. Waddington provided valuable perspectives for the authors.

Special contributions were made by MGMA Human Resources Society members, including:

Maureen A. Moran, personnel director, DeKalb Clinic Chartered, DeKalb, Ill.; **Jeffrey W. Maida**, director of human resources, Duluth Clinic Ltd., Duluth, Minn.; **William C. Stricker**, director of human resources, Wichita Clinic, P.A., Wichita, Kan.

In addition, these MGMA members provided insights into their performance management approaches:

Elaine Raines, director of personnel & clinic services, McFarland Clinic, Ames, Iowa; **Diana Shaw**, Department of Urology, Rochester University, Rochester, N.Y.; and **Grace Hodgson**, office manager, Satterfield, Haakenson, Henderson, Raleigh, N.C.

The importance of performance management

Chapter One

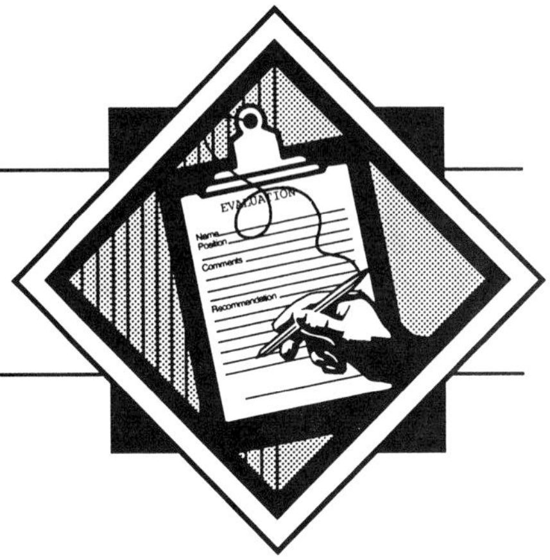

Consultants frequently tell about a classic case of performance "management." It goes like this. One day a consultant was asked by a CEO to visit his organization and advise him about a problem performer. After spending a considerable amount of time listening to the CEO complain about how the subordinate never did what was expected, the consultant asked to see the employee's job description. The CEO pulled it out of his desk for the consultant to review. After studying it for a few minutes, the consultant said, "This seems to be perfectly clear. Did the person have any questions when you discussed this with him?" The CEO replied, "I didn't show it to him. This is my document. He is just expected to know what to do." Then the CEO excused himself to attend to a conference call. While he was gone, the consultant put the job description in a file folder and walked down to talk with the employee. He asked, "What do you think the problem is?" The employee said, "I just can't figure out what he expects from me." The consultant said, "I need to go to my car and get something. While I am gone, you might like to take a look at what is in this file folder." When

he returned, he took back the folder and put the description back on the CEO's desk. Later he suggested to the CEO that they give the matter a few days. When he called the following week and asked how things were going, the CEO said, "I can't understand it. It's like a miracle. All of a sudden the employee is right on target. He is a very successful performer!"

> “We are on the cutting edge — in the talking stage. Right now we are back with the pack, at the point of a rating system where you check the box. There are just pockets of hope that indicate we are moving forward.”
>
> *(MGMA member, medium-sized clinic)*

No matter what it is called — performance appraisal, performance evaluation, performance rating, performance review, performance assessment, performance planning — the performance management process is a vital aspect of human resource management. It can eliminate performance misunderstandings between supervisors and employees. It can make the difference when facing present and future productivity and profitability challenges.

To ensure success for organizations and employees, there is increased focus today on identifying performance expectations upfront, reinforcing them consistently and rewarding results regularly. Medical practices, like other organizations in the health care field, have a particular impetus for focusing on an effective performance management process (PMP).

Society is demanding that health care providers have systems that result in productivity and cost consciousness. Competitors on the total quality management bandwagon are getting the kind of employee performance that is needed to deliver the quality service expected by today's health care customers. In short, to maintain and expand their customer and financial base, medical practices need a performance management process that is contemporary, easy to administrate — and that works!

There has always been a focus on quality assurance in health care; it is a primary fact of life in such organizations. However, now there is an even more intense effort on measuring the quality of work of all workers, not just the caregivers. The quality of performance, whether of a physician or nurse or receptionist, is on the line. As customer expectations get higher and higher, total quality performance management becomes more vital. Indeed, quality assurance and the extent to which quality of work can be measured are growing concerns in all areas of health care.

PERFORMANCE MANAGEMENT USES

"Performance management" is useful terminology for the process since such terms as "performance appraisal" imply a judgmental role rather than a developmental or improvement role. Such phrases also suggest an after-the-fact approach to dealing with employee performance. Current philosophies and management styles place greater emphasis on the upfront need to develop and improve the knowledge, skills, abilities and experiences of employees at all levels in an organization on a consistent basis. "Process" is also useful terminology since it conveys the idea of constant communication throughout the work year rather than a once-a-year discrete event.

In conjunction with this trend is the necessity to encourage improved performance by involving employees in developing and managing their performance plans from the day they start and throughout their careers with the organization. Medical practice administrators now realize that this type of two-way communication with frequent feedback results in the kind of highly motivated and skilled work force that is critical to organizational success today.

Not only is the performance management process an integral part of productivity, but also it is a source of the critical data needed for planning, managing, innovating and reacting to a constantly changing marketplace. Data about performance levels is required generally for staffing, training and placement decisions, and specifically for wage and salary administration, promotions, demotions, transfers and termination decisions.

Performance management systems also are crucial in protecting organizations against legal suits by employees who have been disciplined, fired or adversely affected by management actions.

Poor performance management processes all too often becomes a medical practice's Achilles' heel. Typical example: A supervisor ignores a sensitive performance situation for many months, and neglects to counsel the employee about the problems and to document them. One day the supervisor fires the employee — and the organization gets hit with a suit that it will very likely lose since previous years of performance evaluation all document that the employee had been an above average performer.

Lastly, effective performance management processes have become increasingly important because of the "pay for performance" trend being implemented in many organizations. Compensating employees according to their performance requires that a valid and defensible performance management process be established and maintained.

Figure 1.1

Current dilemmas

Medical practices today are facing the challenge of scrutinizing their performance management process in terms of:

- the objectives they have;
- the tools/forms they use;
- the administrative system they implement; and
- the procedures they promote.

CURRENT DILEMMAS

Ideally, performance management is both a system of communication and a partnership between the supervisor and the employee. Unfortunately, few organizations have ideal processes. Thus, present methods need to be scrutinized from several angles. (See Figure 1.1)

Often performance evaluation problems stem from the:

- appraisal tool itself;
- objective it is intended to serve;
- administrative system in which it is embedded;
- required forms and procedures;
- desire of supervisors to have a quick and easy process with little or no input from employees; and
- scant attention given to training supervisors about the system or on handling the process in a consistent, fair manner.

Most important, many performance evaluation forms are inadequate and:

- not specific;
- not job related;
- not objective;
- not evaluative rather than judgmental;

- not focused on performance improvement and developmental planning;
- not related to the mission or goals of the organization; and
- not clear about what "success" looks like.

Finally, few meet the legal requirements of a defensible system or conform to equal employment legislation. The end result of all these system failures is that the process becomes a joke, a meaningless ritual that erodes the confidence of employees in management.

Most important, research noted in a recent issue of *The Health Care Supervisor* indicated that less than 50 percent of the organizations surveyed use performance evaluation as a means of improving performance which is one of the primary goals of evaluating performance.[1]

Other studies show that as few as 25 percent of employees know what they will be evaluated on before the evaluation takes place. For the majority, the traditional end-of-the-year annual review represents unpleasant surprises, bad news or disappointment.[2]

It is no surprise then to learn that other surveys show that most employees indicate that they believe that performance review sessions do not give them a clear picture of what is expected, what they are doing wrong or how they could improve or advance in the organization. Only half indicate that their bosses help them set performance objectives and only a few say their performance reviews were followed up during the year afterward.[3]

Key problems

Often managers have inappropriate, and even counterproductive beliefs about why organizations have performance evaluations. Much of this misunderstanding occurs because organizations have poorly designed systems that focus on judging the employee as a person — rather than on evaluating job performance and behavior. As a result, performance interviews often reflect a parent-child relationship — an awkward situation that causes tension and distress for both the employee and supervisor.

In addition, many organizations inadequately invest in the performance management process in terms of:

- developing a philosophy about performance management;
- integrating performance management into strategic planning;
- building an organizational chart keyed to performance;
- updating job analyses/descriptions;
- developing performance standards;
- preparing the organization for implementation;
- training and educating supervisors and employees;
- developing performance plans with each employee;
- ensuring ongoing monitoring of performance;
- insisting on frequent and fair evaluations;
- dealing with performance problems quickly and effectively;
- rewarding employees appropriately for successful performance; and
- updating the system as situations change.

Organizations particularly tend to poorly define criteria for what constitutes effective levels of performance. They fail to encourage and provide for self-evaluation by the employee. And they tie the performance process to administrative issues, such as compensation, rather than to the development of the employee, the supervisor and the organization.

Most important, they neglect follow-up. Administrators may have an appropriate process and have implemented it well — but it becomes something to do sometime and never happens. Soon employees recognize it's not real and do what they have always done, which typically is not on target and not as successful as it could be.

Figure 1.2

Effective vs. ineffective performance management process

An **effective** process results in improved:

- communication;
- self-confidence;
- planning;
- staffing;
- personal satisfaction;
- employee development;
- documentation;
- compensation link;
- performance; and
- productivity.

An **ineffective** process results in decreased:

- accountability;
- job satisfaction;
- organizational commitment;
- job knowledge;
- employee loyalty;
- supervisor progress; and
- litigation success.

In health care organizations, this lack of follow-up is often justified as the result of "a greater need." That is, the critical nature of health care puts such a strong emphasis on treating patients that improving the ability of employees to do that work is not seen as equally important — or given much thought at all.

Performance management benefits

For the organization, an effective performance management process allows an organization to set compensation rates, select employees for training programs and prepare promising employees to meet anticipated staffing needs. Properly conducted, performance discussions can help build morale and improve productivity.

For the individual, an effective performance management process informs the employee about the job performance criteria — the basis for evaluation. Properly conducted performance discussions provide employees with help in attaining the expected level of performance and assistance in further development of personal skills in terms of increased knowledge, better human relations skills and potential career growth. They also lead to appropriate rewards for contributions and provide motivation for future performance. (See Figure 1.2)

Employees want and expect a performance process to:

- help them improve in their jobs;
- aid them in achieving their career goals;
- evaluate them fairly on job related performance factors;
- clarify their supervisors' performance expectations; and
- help determine appropriate changes in salary and position.

Managers want and expect a performance process to result in:

- enhanced communication;
- increased employee self-confidence;
- better planning;
- improved staffing;
- increased employee job satisfaction;
- more attention to employee development;
- improved documentation;
- better linkage to compensation;
- enhanced performance; and
- increased productivity.

Inadequate performance processes

In contrast, a poor performance management process results in:

- lower productivity;
- decreased employee satisfaction;
- less organizational commitment;
- poor job understanding;
- less focused planning;
- more turnover;
- decreased likelihood of recognizing above standard performance;
- unwarranted disciplinary actions;
- increased likelihood of conflict with supervisor; and
- higher potential for litigation.

No medical practice can afford such results. Therefore, investing a reasonable amount of time and effort in developing and maintaining an effective performance management process will bring a positive return.

Performance management is management

A key insight into the importance of performance management is gained by focusing on the word "management." Performance management is what management is all about; that is, supervisors plan, organize, lead and control performance. An effective performance management process enhances each of those tasks and results in improved productivity. Supervisors are expected to have foresight about what is needed, to plan how to achieve those goals, to organize work efforts appropriately, to lead workers in the right direction and to monitor and control performance so it stays on target.

> "Performance management is a matter of building relationships, a partnership. Partners need to know what's important, what are the priorities. Everyone needs input in a work setting, such as partners do in a marriage, in a family."
>
> *(MGMA member, large clinic)*

Dialogue is the key to this success. By communicating with employees from start to finish about goals and expectations, supervisors are much more likely to have successful results. Their communication must be true communication — two-way between the supervisor and employee. Unless there is dialogue before starting down the performance path together, supervisors will lack the ideas and information that employees have, and never gain their interest, involvement or investment in the results.

An effective performance management process provides periodic opportunities for communication between the person who assigns the work and the person who performs it. The supervisor has a chance to communicate clearly where the organization wants to go as well as where the employee stands with the organization. The employee has the opportunity to point out barriers to success, such as inadequate resources or unexpected new assignments, and to ask for help with skill development.

A properly designed performance management process is based on comprehensive job analyses and job descriptions that identify critical performance factors and performance standards. These criteria are then used to evaluate how well the employee is meeting the standards. When individuals perform well, they should be rewarded in the form of merit raises, bonuses, promotion opportunities and other benefits in proportion to the contribution they make to the growth and health of the organization.

The principle that should guide a medical practice's performance process is fairness. The organization must recognize that there is a performance-reward cycle — employees perform as expected if they are rewarded as expected, and then they will perform successfully again. Employees also expect that managers are committed to accepting responsibility for carrying out each step of the performance management process in a thorough and consistent way, yet flexible enough to adjust to the dynamics of the organization and the changing world.

Summing up

An effective performance management process can motivate employees to do their best. Success for supervisors is optimum employee performance. This is the only way health care organizations will fulfill their goals in today's competitive environment and develop their employees in ways that lead to both organizational and individual growth.

Medical practice managers can use a performance management process to serve several purposes:

- motivate and retain employees;
- reinforce exceptional performance;
- recognize and reward outstanding employees;
- identify and develop substandard employees;
- comply with the requirements of the Joint Commission on Accreditation of Healthcare Organization; and
- monitor compliance with the Equal Employment Opportunity laws and other court decisions.

The impetus for developing a superior and effective performance management process in a health care organization is very clear. As Charles Joiner wrote, health care organizations are "so employee intensive that salaries and wages comprise as much as 60 to 70 percent of the institution's total operating cost." He notes, this reveals "a clear linkage between the successful operation of the organization and the effective and efficient performance of its employees. A good system can help the organization attract and retain highly qualified employees. Health administrators should clearly understand the reasons for implementing a performance system that is effective in promoting organizational goals as well as in developing human resources."[4]

Footnotes

[1]*William Umiker, M.D. "Performance Review Interviews: Planning for the Future,"* The Health Care Supervisor, *March 1992, p. 29.*

[2]*Patricia King.* Performance Planning & Appraisal. *McGraw-Hill Book Company, New York, 1989.*

[3]*Paul Preston, Ph.D. "Reducing Conflict in Performance Appraisal,"* Administrative Radiology, *November 1991, p. 44.*

[4]*Charles L. Joiner. "Performance Appraisal,"* Strategic Management of Human Resources in Health Services Organizations. *Wiley Medical Books, 1988, p. 319.*

Contemporary performance management processes

Chapter Two

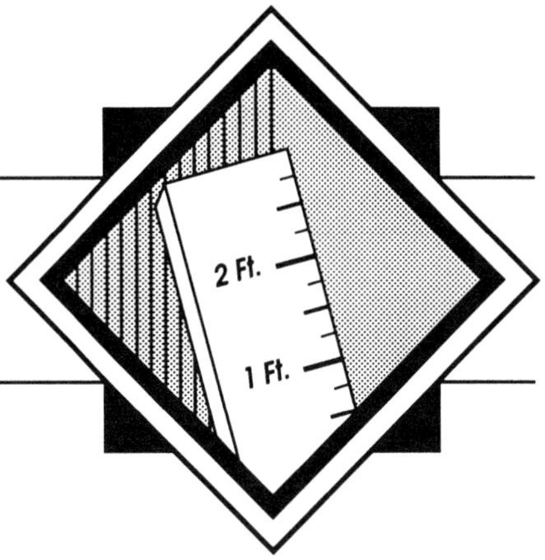

A health care organization that has been using total quality management for five years has completely changed its performance evaluation system. Instead of using its traditional forms and reviewing/rewarding individual performance at a year-end conference conducted by the supervisor, it relies on an "annual piece of paper." At the beginning of each year, the supervisor and employee sit down and discuss how the employee would like to develop this year and how the supervisor/organization can help. The focus is completely developmental. Performance goals are identified and implemented by quality teams that are formed as opportunities for improvement are chosen. Rewards/profits are shared equally. Salaries are based on competitive market surveys and cost-of-living and are not directly linked to individual performance.

Performance evaluation has always been part of life because of a natural need to know "how we are doing." In the work world, such appraisal has ranged from unconscious to informal to quite deliberate and sophisticated.

The evolution of performance management continues today. In fact, it is now in considerable flux as the nation scrambles to find new and better ways to improve productivity — a major challenge for all organizations, including medical practices. This evolution will never end because the world will keep changing and new knowledge will be gained about humans and performance. There will always be a new twist, like total quality management, on its way.

History of performance management

Some things, however, will not change. For one, human beings are measuring animals. From the beginning of time, they have compared themselves with their own past performance and with the performance of others. They would ask, "How many bison did you kill today? Was it more than yesterday? Was it more than Joe?"

Humans also realized that some sort of "return" came from performance evaluation. A court jester knew his performance would be evaluated by the king, and the result would be a kick or a coin. These days, the questions are the same, "What is your golf handicap? Did you improve it today? Was your score better than Joe's?" "Did you get the trophy or the booby prize?"

This normal human need to measure, compare and compensate has always been true in the work world as well. Supervisors forever and ever have made judgments about job performance — based on some yardstick in their heads. Supervisors always have a perception of "what counts" and often it is uniquely personal. The decision about evaluation and "rewards" is often very subjective.

Co-workers also make judgments. Individuals invariably evaluate one another, and they certainly do so in their daily work relationships. Each person judges others' work constantly. However, these judgments may not be logical or communicated.

This type of informal, mostly unconscious method of evaluation was the norm until the industrial revolution. As factory assembly lines became the standard mode of operation, standards were set in a mechanistic, quantifiable way; i.e., amount of time taken to pound a nail, number of items produced in a certain time frame, number of motions used to perform a certain task. However, little consideration was given to the environmental or motivational conditions that influence performance. And rewards were typically based on arbitrary management decisions.

Psychological imperatives

By the 1930s, industrial psychologists began to work with industrial engineers to focus on some of these influencing conditions. The classic Hawthorne plant studies at Western Electric, on the effects of providing an opportunity to talk about work conditions, demonstrated how paying attention to human needs resulted in improved performance.[1]

Other studies verified the premise that humans need to feel useful and valuable. Work provides that opportunity and employers can provide acknowledgment of value received. Work for pay just to provide for the survival and safety motivational needs was necessary. However, as Abraham Maslow illustrated in his classic hierarchical model of needs (See Figure 2.1), work also fulfilled social,

Figure 2.1

Maslow's human motivation model

Abraham Maslow identified a hierarchy of five basic human needs: survival, safety, social, self-esteem, self-actualization.

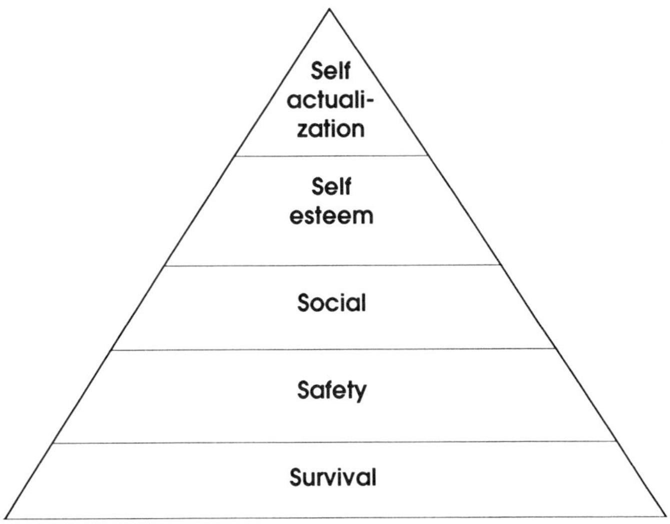

Based on Maslow's human motivation model.

self-esteem and self-actualization needs. It made a person part of a group and "appropriate" performance allowed a person to feel important in that group.[2]

Other psychologists, such as Frederick Herzberg, clarified the motivational importance of hygiene factors that are extrinsic to the job, such as: supervision, interpersonal relationships, working conditions, salary and status. These factors are expected by employees and, therefore, have little motivational value. (See Figure 2.2)

Figure 2.2

Herzberg motivational factors

Frederick Herzberg divided motivational factors into dissatisfiers/hygiene factors (supervision, interpersonal relationships, working conditions, compensation, status) and satisfiers/motivators (work itself, responsibility, advancement, growth, achievement).

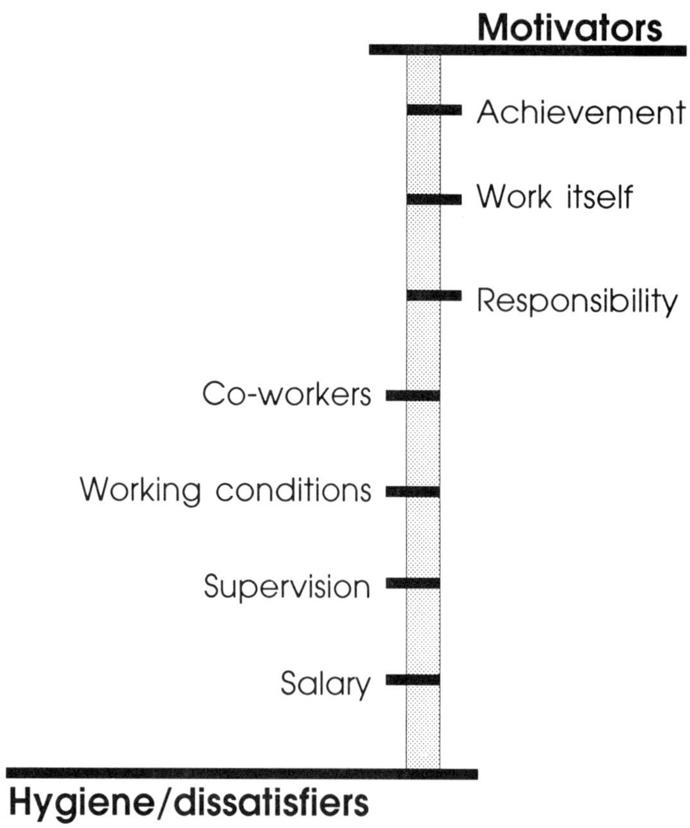

Based on Herzberg's motivation model.

In contrast, he found that the key motivators are intrinsic and relate to: the work itself, responsibility, advancement, growth, achievement. These factors "turn on" workers.[3]

This is the area of self-actualization — of reaching one's self-potential. As Maslow said, "What a man can be, he must be." It is natural for humans to strive to be all they can be.

Psychologists recognized the connection of this need to measurement. They confirmed that the very act of measuring, influences the behavior of the people being measured. When supervisors measure employees' performance, they create a motivational ripple effect.

Employees tend to interpret the measurements as defining important aspects of the job. They respond by trying to "hit the mark" at a level that will be rewarded. In other words, when employees know what "counts" — what results in increased productivity and rewards — they see a new value in productivity.[4]

These behavioral psychologists also discovered that a higher level of achievement motivation occurs when the goals are stretch goals — realistic yet ambitious. Challenging goals stimulate reasonable risk-taking and higher performance. Most important, ongoing motivation occurs if supervisors give employees feedback on how they are doing in achieving goals.

These psychological basics continue to be highly relevant today. When examined for their behavioral implications, performance planning and measurements have a major impact on how managers make their influence felt. Planning and goal setting can be loaded with motivational triggers that encourage self-responsibility, moderate risk-taking and achievement-oriented behavior.

In addition, performance goals can stimulate collaborative and cooperative behavior. Performance expectations and feedback signal that certain behaviors are valued and others are not. By skillfully using these concepts, management can move organizations forward significantly.[5]

> "Rather than a performance report card, there is a movement toward dialog, a partnership between supervisor and employee. Structured facilitation is emphasized rather than a parent-child approach in terms of what needs to be done, what the employee wants to do and how we are going to get there. TQM is the driving force for this change.
>
> "However, I still don't see any clear direction for performance management. There is a lot of evaluation bashing today, especially by TQM advocates. But there are no good solutions yet; we just know the current situation doesn't work. We are all in search of the new Holy Grail."
>
> *(MGMA member, medium-sized clinic)*

Tool development

Although these concepts have been known for several decades, they were not quickly applied in the form of methods and tools that did indeed promote performance goal and standard setting or monitoring and feedback. The fact is that employee performance evaluation is a relatively primitive administrative art. Even sophisticated, mature organizations tend to be dissatisfied with their methods for appraising and improving employee performance. The concept of one person judging another fosters a feeling of discomfort and results in ineffectiveness.

That was certainly an accurate perception of the early tools. First-generation performance review tools typically were a checklist of personality traits in a report card format. Supervisors assessed such characteristics as cooperativeness, adaptability, dependability, appearance and attitude based on an evaluation scale that gave no clues about what these factors were — or what effect they had on performance.[6]

The system based an employee's entire rating on personality judgments. Supervisors and employees only discussed the review if individuals complained about the "grades." Not only was this a backward look at performance, but performance was not job related, defined or measured in results.

An improvement on this approach came in the 1960s with the introduction of management by objectives. This forward looking approach emphasized interviews between supervisors and employees during which goals were negotiated and quantified. However, although what was to be counted was clear, often little attention was given to other critical factors, such as time and resources allocated, and often goals were not modified as situations changed. Management by objectives was usually reserved for professional and management staff.

The next phase focused on systems still in use today that are based on the employee's job description rather than personality assessment. This was an important advance. However, this task-based approach typically uses five to six subjective assessments that range from "awful" to "wonderful" to appraise performance. Frequently, there are few clues about what is unsatisfactory, marginal, satisfactory, superior, outstanding performance.

A more recent move has been to tools that define specific tasks, goals and responsibilities that can be measured in objective terms. They also must identify specific criteria that can be assessed against a standard of quality, quantity, cost and/or timeliness. In sum, contemporary performance management tools aim to:

- clarify job expectations;
- facilitate upfront mutual goal-setting by the supervisor and employee and development of realistic performance standards;
- promote ongoing monitoring and correction by both the supervisor and employee; and
- provide final evaluations that summarize not only results but also what has been learned and can be used in the future. This discussion essentially provides the groundwork for the next cycle of planning.

The main goal is to objectively measure and improve performance. A strong secondary goal is to develop the employee. Effective performance management plans must be a “win-win” for both the employee and the organization.

Inherent in this process is ensuring that the system has the objectivity, validity and legal defensibility required for effective compensation systems, promotions, employee redeployment or termination. Work evaluations are behaviorally or criterion-based and the performance standards are keyed to job description duties and strategic plan objectives.

Practical imperatives

More and more organizations, including medical practices, are moving to contemporary systems because of a series of recent events that have stimulated change. The first is a heightened awareness of employment law and regulations and their potential not just for punishment — but for performance. Civil rights and equal employment opportunity laws were revised and strengthened during the middle 1960s, but it took many years for organizations to recognize that these requirements affect job performance and motivation.

Requiring current job descriptions based on thorough job analysis, development of job-related criteria, periodic measurement of performance and assistance for inadequate performance results in a clear focus on "what success is." With such information, an organization can select better and manage better. It will also help them identify and take disciplinary action on employees whose performance fails to improve.

The second event is the change in the values of employees. Workers now expect to be involved in work plans and decisions that affect them. This new mindset puts the spotlight on employee rights, all the way from negotiating their own goals, expecting feedback and fair evaluations, and knowing there should be a fair appeal process and consistent management oversight of the process.

Third is the escalation of human resource costs. As America becomes more and more of a service industry country, employees become the biggest line item in the budget.

Organizations cannot afford to mismanage them. It must choose them wisely and guide their performance thoughtfully. "Our people are our most important assets" is a common bottom line, hard core economic theme today.

The fourth event is the national focus on productivity. As European and Japanese companies passed the United States in the productivity race, American organizations began to pay more attention to the management practices that caused these results. Of particular interest were Japanese styles of management that focus on employee involvement and commitment to performance improvement. Competitively, this nation now knows it must find new answers.[7]

Self assessment

Some of the performance management methods being promoted today actually have been around for a while,

> “TQM is part of what's prompting us to change our performance system. We know that if we want the employee group to respond, we must have upward involvement — not just downward. We'd like the employee to take initiative and responsibility for the bottom line.
>
> "CQI is an issue for all industries. It is becoming more and more critical for group practices. We started our CQI initiative three years ago. At that time we had a traditional performance appraisal/merit pay system. Through a long educational process, we have changed our approach to performance review completely. We now have many feedback forms that managers use to get additional input for performance reviews. These are for use by peers, co-workers, customers, peer-supervisors, supervisors to employees. During the performance review the supervisor uses all the feedback. Self-appraisal is another option.”
>
> *(MGMA member, large city clinic)*

but are being seen in a new positive light. One of the most valuable is self-evaluation, or more broadly known today as self-management or self-responsibility.

Many studies have shown that ratings of employees themselves are often more accurate than those done by supervisors. Inflation bias of course can occur in self-evaluation. However, as long as the success target is perfectly clear and they are rewarded for communicating mistakes as well as successes, employees are highly likely to evaluate themselves honestly.[8]

This employee-driven approach gained significant impetus from the recent restructuring and downsizing efforts of many organizations. As lean and mean companies began asking for more performance from fewer employees, they not only had to target desired outcomes precisely, but also to count on employees to manage their own performance. The best use of fewer managers is to help employees plan performance and to coach them to success, provide a supportive environment — and let them run with the ball.

There is a Catch-22 for the employee in this approach, however. There has been a deterioration of a time honored, unwritten but implicitly understood contract between organization and employee: “Do a good job and you will have a job.” Organizations can no longer honor this agreement. Because of the economy, mergers and competition, no medical practice is protected from the possibility of downsizing or even of closure.[9]

The challenge then becomes to promote self-responsibility and effective performance as even more essential to employees. The message is three-fold:

- When you do your best, we have a much better chance of surviving and your keeping your job.
- If you lose your job, you will take with you an excellent performance record, strong recommendations and enhanced knowledge, skills and abilities that are your best career assets.
- Psychologically humans feel better about themselves when they, managing their performance, perform well.

Self-management involves full participation in planning and setting goals and equal responsibility with the supervisor for monitoring and correcting performance. Employees are expected to:

- take the initiative to alert the supervisor of problems or mistakes;
- suggest corrective solutions;
- formally assess their performance, using a self-evaluation tool, at specified times; and
- compare the self-assessment with their supervisor's assessment.

If the two have been working in partnership during the performance period, the evaluations should be very similar. If not, the two must analyze why the discrepancies occurred and how to eliminate them in the future.

Peer evaluation

Co-worker evaluation generally shows greater consistency than supervisor ratings for these reasons:

- It uses a multiple rater system. The perspectives of several people provide a more comprehensive view of performance;
- Co-workers have the opportunity to observe a fellow employee's behavior more closely and more frequently. They see the patterns of appropriate or inappropriate behaviors and are much less likely to have their evaluation influenced by an occasional deviation; and
- They are much more likely to understand the environmental and motivational conditions impacting the employee. Peers, of course, are just as susceptible to biases as other raters. Therefore, the rating system must use objective standards of measurement.

Co-workers may feel awkward, or even afraid, about doing peer ratings, especially if their evaluations are negative. Therefore, it is essential to build protection into the system for employee and peers by following these guidelines:

> “Fighting TQM is like fighting Mom and apple pie. It is nothing new; it's always been needed. To get it started, you need a cheerleader. Long-term employees struggle more with it because it appears as just one more thing.”
>
> *(MGMA member, small, rural clinic)*

- Management must carefully communicate with employees about the purpose of such a system and how they will be involved;
- Rating data should be kept anonymous, gathered by a neutral party, consolidated into group results and presented privately to the employee; and
- The employee should be encouraged to work with his/her supervisor on particular performance areas seen as needing improvement by the group.

Peer ratings have been used for some time in some professional circles, including health care professionals such as physicians. Again, the premise is that those who do certain tasks are the best qualified to evaluate others who do the same tasks.

Staff evaluation

In health care organizations, as in other businesses, it is standard practice to seek staff input when gathering performance data about an employee. Example: A nurse may report to a nursing supervisor, but is assigned to work with one or more physicians. These physicians are then asked to evaluate the nurse from their perspective.

Professional staff input can be handled most effectively by focusing on:

- **time requirements**. Physicians have little time, or patience, for dealing with more paperwork. Thus, using a tool that is quick to complete is vital; and
- **objectivity requirements**. Physicians like all human beings can easily fall into the subjective judgment trap unless they are provided with objective measurement tools. Having physicians participate in the process of establishing performance standards is a most useful step. This involvement will help them understand how a process based on job-related criteria works and will stimulate them to be effective in observing and reporting performance in specific behavioral terms.

Manager evaluation

Managers are also occasionally evaluated by peers. However, the nontraditional approach gaining most favor for management evaluation is employee evaluation of supervisors. Although this may be a threatening idea for some managers, today it is seen as a very valuable way to help supervisors become more effective.

Employees have the best view of the effects of their supervisors. They know how it impacts them and their performance. They are often more accurate at rating their managers than the managers are at rating themselves.

To ensure the system is just as fair and objective for managers as for employees, the information collected must be job related, not personality-based. Having supervisors and employees identify the dimensions to be evaluated and the appropriate rating system is a necessary step.

Again, anonymity must be guaranteed for those who provide feedback. The results should be consolidated by a neutral party, such as the person responsible for human resource matters. The results then should go directly to the supervisor, who should be encouraged to share them with his or her manager to work on improvement areas identified by employees.

Like any individual receiving feedback, supervisors may respond constructively to upward evaluations and begin to change behaviors, or they may become depressed or angry. To ensure a positive response, senior management must provide the appropriate context, training and support. The focus: improved performance, not punishment.[10]

Upward evaluations often lead to better working relationships between supervisors and employees — and thus to higher productivity. For example, if employees rate their supervisor poorly on communication, the supervisor can work on improving this skill.

An excellent approach is to have the supervisor do a self-assessment and to compare it with the employees' assessment. The insights gained from any discrepancies are very enlightening. They should be discussed with both the supervisor's subordinates and his or her manager.

Another variation that can be used is to have the supervisor ask for staff input by completing an evaluation or similar form that the supervisor can use in planning his or her own development plans. Employees usually welcome the opportunity to give their evaluation and recommendations for improvement.

Executive evaluation

Developing performance plans and reviewing results for top management, and particularly the chief executive officer, president or executive director, is also being given more attention these days. One reason is the increasing criticism about executive compensation. In both the for-profit and nonprofit worlds there is much controversy about the value of senior management, particularly when pay does not seem to correlate with organizational performance.

Hence, there is renewed interest in determining what executive performance should be. For example:

- Is the CEO's evaluation based on astute strategic planning and fulfillment of long-term goals, and/or on short-run achievements?
- Does the CEO have the necessary knowledge, skills and abilities to lead the organization into the future?
- Does the CEO demonstrate leadership in terms of visionary planning and empowerment of others?
- Does the CEO recruit, manage and develop an effective staff?
- Who should manage the CEO? Is the board of directors effective?

These are all questions that should be asked and answered. In any case, the executive's performance expectations should be made clear by the board when he or she takes the position. Thereafter, expectations should be planned at the beginning of the fiscal year so they are in sync with the annual work plan/budget and long-range plans.

This performance plan should be negotiated and both personal performance targets and organizational targets identified. Throughout the year, just like any other employee, the CEO should monitor and report on results and make appropriate corrections, as approved by the board. End results should reflect overall achievement for the organization as well as personal achievement.

Often long-term performance objectives are built into an employment contract between the board and the CEO. In addition, compensation/rewards are usually specified in the contract.

CLIENT EVALUATION

An increasingly critical component of medical practice evaluation is patient or customer satisfaction. Having a service centered approach to providing patient care has been the trend in recent years. This movement recognizes changing marketplace values: consumers and payers are shopping around more for health care providers and the deciding factor often is service.

This switch from the perspective of an individual as a patient who is "taken care of" by the provider to a customer with specific service expectations has been quite an adjustment for some physicians and group practices. Even the idea of thinking of an individual as a client has been difficult for some. Nevertheless, most medical practice managers well understand that the real challenge is to convert service concepts into actual on-the-job performance.

The performance management system is a powerful tool for this conversion. Service performance expectations can be incorporated into the performance plan, along with specific descriptions of "what successful service looks like" and how it will be measured.

Some medical practices are far along the client evaluation route; that is, they survey clients consistently. A typical survey asks very specific performance behavior questions that can range from questions about the physician's performance to the pharmacist's to the receptionist's. (See Figure 2.3)

Figure 2.3

Customer satisfaction survey

Many medical practices are surveying customer satisfaction on a regular basis. Such surveys should ask specific behavioral questions.

Examples:

1. Was your medication ready for pickup when the pharmacy said it would be?
2. Did the physician explain the possible side effects of the medications you are taking?
3. Did you have to wait more than 10 minutes in the reception area?

Since the questions are always about observable behaviors, the answers are objective. Examples: "Did the doctor explain your condition in terms you understand? Did the pharmacist go over the dosage instructions with you? When you called to make an appointment, did the receptionist answer your call within three rings?"

One example: The Kaiser Permanente clinics in Denver regularly send out surveys to clients. The surveys are returned to a research firm that tallies the scores and sends the results after about 100 surveys have been received. All of the written comments are sent verbatim. Each department receives its averaged scores. The department manager gives the staff information and resources for improving their art of medicine skills.[11]

Kaiser reports that the feedback has helped. Scores have improved by several points in every area. Other practices have found that this type of "service marketing" clarifies client expectations and enhances clients' perceptions of practice performance.

Team performance

Team building and performance improvement are high priority goals for many medical practices today. An organizational commitment to team building can help managers to fully utilize the organization's human resources and create significant change over time. By developing a performance management process based on specific performance standards related to teamwork, medical practices will benefit from such results as improved goal-setting and problem-solving and increased productivity.

"Team building" is a phrase that can have several meanings. In the contemporary sense it means improving group performance through focus on a common mission, clarified relationships and shared leadership. Two specific applications of today's type of team building are self-managing work teams and multi-skilled teams.

Self-managing teams are another product of the restructuring trend. As organizations reorganize, they often replace many middle managers with teams of line workers. The amount of responsibility and authority given to these teams varies extensively. However, in its ultimate form, self-managing work teams set their own goals in collaboration with upper management, select their own team members, establish their own standards, monitor and evaluate their own performance — and make compensation decisions.

The team leader primarily serves as a coach and a resource and is a buffer/communicator with other parts of the organization. To date, work teams have been most effective in organizations where traditional management methods and managers are not solidly entrenched and where the corporate culture is open to change.

Medical practices that still emphasize the physician-centered model rather than a client orientation are not as accepting of the team approach. However, many practices see the merit of a holistic approach to client service and are beginning to share responsibility and power. Innovation teams are one of the major leverage tools in successful entrepreneurial efforts.[12]

Self-managing teams represent a challenge to performance measurement in that the question becomes: what performance is measured ... group or individual? The answer can be one or the other, but is most effective when it is both. Teams should be formed to fulfill certain goals. Their performance then should be measured by the success of the goals and the total team rewarded equally. Incentives should be structured so that the entire team benefits if certain goals are met or exceeded.[13]

However, individual contributions to team success also should be recognized. The problem: How to structure conditions so individual performance can be observable and attributable? One way is to ensure that the tasks performed by the work group are structured so that the outputs of each member become inputs for the others.

Example: A team is put together to publish a report on a certain procedure. Each member is given an assignment to gather specific information. Another member takes this information and drafts a report. Another individual edits the material. The next produces appropriate graphics. Another formats the material for production. The next copies the material and yet another distributes the report. The chain of contribution is clear and the performance standards are clearly specified in terms of quantity, quality and timeliness.

This approach is not always applicable. Sometimes everyone is doing the same thing or everything at once. In these cases, a peer review system can be used since team members will be the best evaluators of others' contributions. As always, such systems must be based on job-related criteria to reduce rater bias.

Multi-skilled teams are also replacing old work systems. This approach involves developing a broader, more flexible workforce through cross-training of employees — teaching them how to do several jobs — and paying them for the variety of skills they master.

Although cross-training has been emphasized previously, only recently has that idea been coupled with teaming. Now organizations are forming "work design" teams of multi-skilled workers who analyze factors affecting their jobs. They consider productivity, quality, safety and customer service as well as their own employee satisfaction and make decisions about how to improve performance.

Members are selected by their peers based on which employees know the most about all the jobs. They meet regularly and obtain feedback from fellow employees on proposals they make. The focus is on business — they discuss if money is being made or lost and the performance corrections needed.[14]

The team approach is tightly tied to the concept of empowerment. This buzz word has become a part of standard management language and appears to be a useful promoter of performance. It's built on Maslow's premise of "being all you can be." Empowerment promotes self-responsibility for setting personal goals and monitoring personal performance with the guidance and assistance of managers.

Total quality management

The concepts of teaming and empowerment are integrated into the total quality management (TQM) and continuous quality improvement (CQI) movements, which are prevalent in many medical practices today. TQM aims to help organizations meet and exceed the expectations of all its customers, both internal and external. CQI facilitates this by focusing on continuous improvement via small, incremental steps. In sum, as performance gets better everyday, so should quality, productivity and customer satisfaction.

These processes are brought to life by cross-functional teams who are empowered to find "opportunities for improvement" within the system. After they examine present procedures to determine the causes of problems, they develop alternative approaches and pilot them. Throughout the process, they involve other employees in providing information and sharing feedback. Result: When the new procedure is implemented, it has been fully tested and endorsed.

This approach to performance improvement has a long history of working well, particularly in other countries such as Japan. Although it can take several years before significant changes and payoffs occur, proponents feel that TQM is a major key to effective performance management since it spotlights today's hottest performance standard — quality. And it encourages employee involvement and management commitment to change.

However, traditional performance processes may hinder total quality management. TQM guru W. Edwards Deming feels that performance evaluations are deadly and are a prime cause of poor quality. His premise: Individual evaluation nurtures rivalry and destroys teamwork. (See Figure 2.4)

Figure 2.4

W. Edwards Deming's TQM concepts

W. Edwards Deming, the guru of total quality management (TQM), feels that traditional performance appraisals:

- negate long-term performance;
- destroy self-esteem;
- invalidate teamwork;
- stymie leadership;
- penalize risk-takers;
- pressure with numbers;
- discourage quality improvements; and
- punish employees for factors outside their control.

Based on Deming's TQM concepts

As a result of this philosophy, some health care organizations implementing TQM/CQI are changing their performance systems. They are focusing more on organization performance targets, across-the-board rewards for achieving goals and personal development discussions.[15]

The basic premise of TQM is that problems are caused by something wrong with the process rather than with the person. The belief: People want to do their best; the system gets in the way. Thus, the TQM approach is to bring people together to identify the problem, analyze the present process, pinpoint causes of the problem, and to suggest and try new approaches. The focus is always on satisfying the customer — whether that is internally (physician, lab staff, billing department) or externally (patient, pay source, accreditation agency). In this approach, the individual is considered to be part of the solution, not the problem, and group performance is key.

Medical practices can learn from the TQM/CQI efforts of hospitals, who were among the first in health care to incorporate this philosophy into their organizations. They typically start with small, team-based process improvement efforts. These projects usually fall into three categories: support services, medical infrastructure and direct patient care. As these efforts establish a success pattern, the next step is to move into extensive training, revamping of reward/salary systems and self-managing teams.[16]

Future possibilities

In the days ahead, performance measurement increasingly may be monitored electronically. This is already occurring in some industries; for example, in airlines where the productivity of reservation clerks is tracked via computer. Hospitals are also using such systems.

For example, the May 1992 issue of *HR Magazine* reports that hospitals, through their Total Patient Care systems, track daily activities including medication orders, billings, inventory, housekeeping, meals and equipment. In doing so, they are also tracking specific activities such as the number of transactions a staff member initiates, amount of time spent, response time and accuracy of efforts.[17]

The practice of accumulating this information is called automated performance measurement or computerized productivity monitoring or work monitoring. Critics call it electronic surveillance. Whatever it is called, the system uses computer programs and software to record, direct or evaluate the work employees perform.

Will such systems take over? Since management information and medical information systems will continue to advance, it can be predicted that performance data will continue to be collected.

How it is used will be one critical question. Others will relate to the use of technology to program performance; that is, making more use of computer-based training to imprint effective behaviors on new employees. On-the-job training is being re-engineered to seek order-of-magnitude improvements in productivity, not incremental change. Electronic performance support tools are being developed that accelerate initial learning and also serve advisory and reference roles.

To complete the performance technology menu are a variety of new software programs that will develop performance systems for organizations. For example, one such system already on the market ("Performance Trak") consists of several modules related to organizational and personal performance. Via a main menu, users can select options and then are asked a series of questions related to work categories/scales. Within each scale are "critical success factors."

Supervisors enter answers about an employee's performance and the computer records, sums and averages them. The results can be printed or grouped with other data to compare work units or individuals over time or to see differences in perceptions of boss and subordinate. The information provides a rich source of data for human resource analysis. It also is a fertile ground of controversy about depersonalized systems.[18]

Summing up

Of all the possibilities ahead for performance management systems, one approach seems to have the most merit. Involving employees in analyzing and improving performance systems will continue to pay off. This tactic can be used successfully whether the medical practice is small or large.

Organizations that bring together employees in focus groups and task forces to discuss their concerns about the present system and to recommend areas of improvement will see results in terms of important links between corporate strategies and individual performance goals. And such future systems should remove many of the confrontational aspects of evaluation and clearly define the manager as a coach and the relationship between manager and employee as a partnership.

Most important, the success of the partnerships will be verified by 360-degree evaluation — performance outcome measures collected from all audiences; supervisors, managers, peers, clients and employees themselves.

Footnotes

[1]*David R. Hampton, Charles E. Summer, Ross A. Webber.* Organizational Behavior and the Practice of Management. *Glenview, Ill.: Scott, Foresman & Co., 1973, p. 371.*

[2]*ibid, p. 4.*

[3]*ibid, p. 372.*

[4]*ibid, p. 531.*

[5]*ibid, p. 535.*

[6]*William Umiker, M.D. "Performance Review Interviews: Planning for the Future,"* The Health Care Supervisor, *March 1992, p. 28.*

[7]*H. John Bernardin, Richard W. Beatty.* Performance Appraisal: Assessing Human Behavior at Work. *Belmont, Calif.: PWS-Kent Publishing Co., 1984, p. 20.*

[8]*Berkeley Rice. "Performance Review: The Job Nobody Likes,"* Psychology Today, *September 1985, p. 28.*

[9]*"Job Performance, Security: Business Paradox of '90s,"* Rocky Mountain News, *October 14, 1992.*

[10]*Scott Warrick. "Supervisor Review Sheds Light on Blind Spots,"* HR Magazine, *June 1992, p. 111.*

[11]*"Quality Health Care,"* Kaiser Permanente Brochure, *1992.*

[12]*Courtney Price, Alys Novak.* Health Care Innovation and Venture Trends. *Albany, N.Y.: Delmar Publishers, Inc., 1992.*

[13]*Val J. Halamandaris. "Empowering People,"* Caring Magazine, *September 1992, p. 35.*

[14]*D. Keith Denton. "Multi-Skilled Teams Replace Old Work Systems,"* HR Magazine, *September 1992, p. 48.*

[15]*Jim M. Graber, Roger E. Breish, Walter E. Breisch. "Performance Appraisals and Deming: A Misunderstanding?,"* Quality Progress, *June 1992, p. 59.*

[16]*Beverly Geber. "Can TQM Cure Health Care?,"* Training, *August 1992, p. 25.*

[17]*Rebecca Grant. "Work Monitored Electronically,"* HR Magazine, *May 1992, p. 81.*

[18]*Paul Slattery. "A New Way to Appraise,"* HR Magazine, *October 1991, p. 27.*

Objectives of performance management

Chapter Three

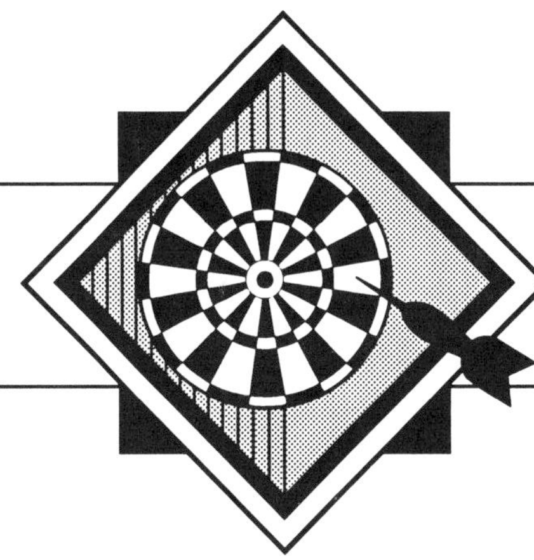

At its annual planning retreat, the managers of a medical practice invited a health care futurist to give them a preview of the future. She described the trends already looming on the horizon — from health care reform initiated by federal and state governments, to technological advances, to dramatic demographic/ psychographic shifts. After the presentation, the managers brainstormed about the type of employee skills they will need in this future where change will be constant, where speed of adjustment will be critical, where hierarchies will be replaced by bubble charts. They decided the "perfect employee" should not only have technical competence, but also should have the skills to adapt quickly, to provide quality customer service, to be accountable, to take initiative, to deal with information effectively, to be self-responsible, to participate fully in multi-skilled, self-managing teams. They also decided they need to change their performance management process to fit the future.

Before a medical group practice begins to develop a new performance management process, or to revise a current one, its managers need to ask themselves a variety of questions:

- What do we have now?
- How is it working?
- What concerns or challenges does it cause?

Then comes the hard question: What should the future system look like? The answer must factor in many variables, including changing times, changing values, changing markets and changing ways of doing business. Most important, the answer must be based on what the managers of the medical practice believe is best for the organization.

As a first objective, management needs to develop a philosophy about performance management. In this case, the questions it must ask include:

- What fits the corporate culture, the organizational climate?
- What has been the historical approach (traditional parent-child, professional peer, laissez-faire, no system at all)?
- Is the present system backward or forward looking?
- Does it evaluate individual or group performance?
- Does it reward short-term or long-term performance?
- Is it job related?
- Does it encourage participation and involvement?
- Does it promote pay-for-performance?
- What values generated support the current system?

It is vital to get these belief systems out on the table because feelings are just as important to consider as facts when analyzing a performance management process and its role as a management tool.

> “The real objective, and value, of a performance review is as a communication tool. It's a communication opportunity. It's an outline for a dialog. The rating piece is a sideline. The focus is on talking with the subordinate about how to improve. The key: the discussion, not the form. The paper is just a reference piece for the discussion and a documentation piece for the files.”
>
> *(MGMA member, large city clinic)*

These beliefs may arise from several sources, including the mission of the organization, whether it is a for-profit or nonprofit corporation, the age of the organization, its size, its employee composition, its client base, its compensation practices, its management style, the values of key players, etc.

Particularly relevant is the age of the organization. As a medical practice evolves from the entrepreneurial startup stage to the growth stage to the maturity stage to the decline stage, its philosophy about performance management often evolves as well. In the early stages, the mood is often "all for one and one for all." There is a strong team spirit, support for each other's performance and sharing of rewards.

As the organization grows into maturity, the organizational climate tends to become more structured with more systems and less flexibility. Individual, immediate contributions may get lost in the focus on long-term results. In the decline stage, a philosophy of "hold it together as long as we can" may prevail. Performance becomes basically a survival game with less and less motivation to improve.

Regardless of the phase or the factors that impact the medical practice, its managers must discuss and establish an updated philosophy on "how we want to do it in the future." This philosophy should be stated openly to employees via the employee manual and other communication modes as part of the explanation of what kind of performance management system the organization has, how it works and how it ties everything together from organizational strategic planning to individual performance planning.

Strategic planning

This philosophy becomes the backdrop for the medical practice's strategic planning. As the practice plans its future, it should remain cognizant of what its managers believe about performance.

Strategic planning is another objective of performance management. This big-picture, long-term planning establishes the performance goals for the organization and sets the scene for employee performance goals.[1]

Strategic planning involves envisioning where the organization should be in the years ahead, and determining how to get there. Such planning is done in the context of looking at both the external and internal environment (present strengths and weaknesses). Of key importance is a trends analysis to identify potential opportunities and threats that may impact the medical practice.

Figure 3.1

Trend analysis technique

Group practices should keep their eye on trends on the horizon using a STEP analysis technique.

❶ **S**ocial; e.g., aging, cultural diversity;

❷ **T**echnological; e.g., genetic engineering, automation;

❸ **E**conomics; e.g., recession, competition; and

❹ **P**olitical; e.g., health care reform, regulation.

This type of analysis is called STEP analysis because it looks at **S**ocial, **T**echnological, **E**conomic and **P**olitical trends. There are always some general trends that will affect all organizations, such as an economic recession, and there will be specific trends that directly impact certain industries. (See Figure 3.1)

Medical practice managers should keep their eyes on the industry's future "hot buttons." (See Figure 3.2 on page 39.) These trend busters range from the aging boom to the baby boomers.[2] For health care providers, major trends include:

- **payment reform**. Primary physicians are facing more competition from "holistic approaches" with outpatient ambulatory practice groups gaining in strength. There will be increasingly competitive situations with hospitals as more physicians set up clinics;
- **demographics**. The baby boomer demographic surge is hitting the health care sector and they will demand more and better services. Boomers are facing their major health care consumption period;
- **the graying of America**. As individuals live longer, the number of frail elderly will increase and cause a severe drain on the social and health care system;
- **exclusive arrangements**. There will be continued turmoil in the provider world between the buyer, the medical seller and the intermediaries, such as insurance companies. Buyers will look at intermediaries more critically and some, such as large corporations, may buy directly from providers;
- **consolidation**. Medical sellers will get more sophisticated. The system of medical care (hospitals, group practices, home health care) will get more integrated. This is already happening in the Midwest where there are very large group practices and mergers of group

practices with hospitals. These sophisticated sellers are beginning to deal directly with large corporate buyers;

- **efficiency**. All health care providers are having to become more efficient, to reduce redundancy, to streamline. They are restructuring how they do business, for example, orienting services into decentralized, patient-service units;
- **quality/customer satisfaction**. More health care organizations are adopting the total quality management approach, including employee involvement and team decision making and customer/marketing orientation;
- **medical information systems**. The collection and utilization of data to guide medical decision-making, internal and external management strategies, and case management has grown increasingly important to medical providers, with associated substantial costs;
- **regulation**. State, federal and private budget constraints are forcing policymakers to seek ways to constrain the growth of health care expenditures. At the same time, providers are obligated to meet the ever-changing standards of care as well as responding to an increasing number of laws and regulations;
- **technology**. Technological innovations from the biomedical and pharmaceutical industries emerge continually, while concerns for utilization and cost effectiveness lead efforts to limit their use. Ethic issues of life and death coincide with these decisions; and
- **universal health care**. Societal pressures have brought the issue of national health care to the forefront of the political arena. Before the end of the decade, some form of mandated health coverage for all Americans is expected.

As medical practices contemplate these trends, they must position themselves in that future and determine where they want to be in that swirling picture. This dream of a desirable future becomes their success target and the driving force for their efforts in the next three to five years

Figure 3.2

Health care hot buttons

Driving forces for the health care sector in the future will be the:

- home health care becoming one of the primary deliveries of health care during the 20th century;
- increasing numbers of those with chronic illness and/or are aging;
- baby boomers who want to live as full and as long a life as possible;
- advances in the high-technology area; e.g., "smart cards," biotechnology, microelectronics, artificial intelligence;
- rural survival dilemma; e.g., decline in agricultural industry stimulating economic innovations;
- continued restructuring of health care delivery from inpatient to outpatient services; and
- adoption of customer-driven marketing and service methods as part of a total quality management philosophy.

Adapted from "Health Care Innovations & Venture Trends"

and, in particular, will identify their annual plan goals. Determining the role of their human resources and how to maximize performance must be part of the equation.

Human resource plan

The next objective is a human resource plan; it should evolve from the strategic plan. It is the natural foundation for policy decisions related to the types of work that must be done to achieve the plan. For example, since marketing is expected to be a prime focus in the years ahead, the medical practice must consider how to best utilize marketing functions and what this means not only in terms of specific jobs, but more important, in terms of marketing training for all staff.

As quality assurance procedures blend into quality management processes, identifying who will make it happen will become more critical. As management and medical information systems become more complex, this function must gain stature in the human resource plan.

In short, once the medical practice decides where it wants to be in the future, it must identify what functions and types of staff this will involve and what processes will be used to recruit, select, train, manage and handle performance planning and evaluation.

For example, if a clinic decides its best future bet is becoming a center of excellence in a certain specialty, such as arthritis, it will need a human resource plan that provides effective staff and systems to fulfill that vision.

Organizational chart

The human resource and strategic plan are the tools for building an organizational chart. The charts of the future may look different than the standard hierarchy of boxes. There is already experimentation with "bubble charts" that show a solid center (the CEO's spot) surrounded by bubbles which represent constantly changing, client-oriented teams or projects. (See Figure 3.3 on page 41)

As one project is finished, the team members scatter and join up with others in a new bubble dedicated to another

Figure 3.3

Organizational chart vs. bubble chart

The classic hierarchical organization chart differs dramatically from today's bubble organizational model.

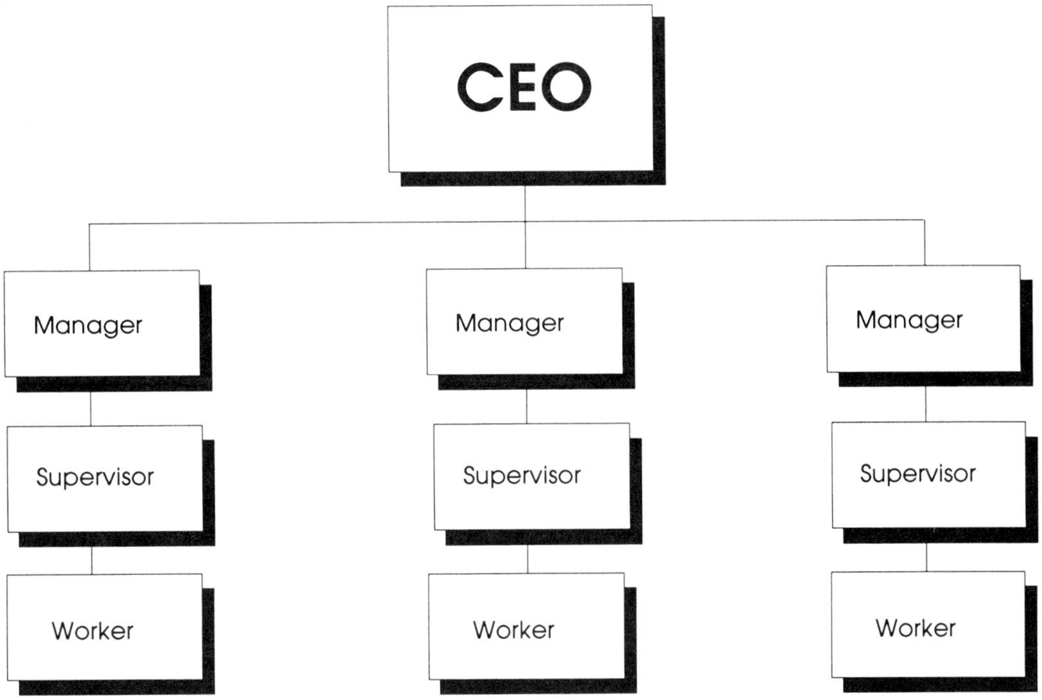

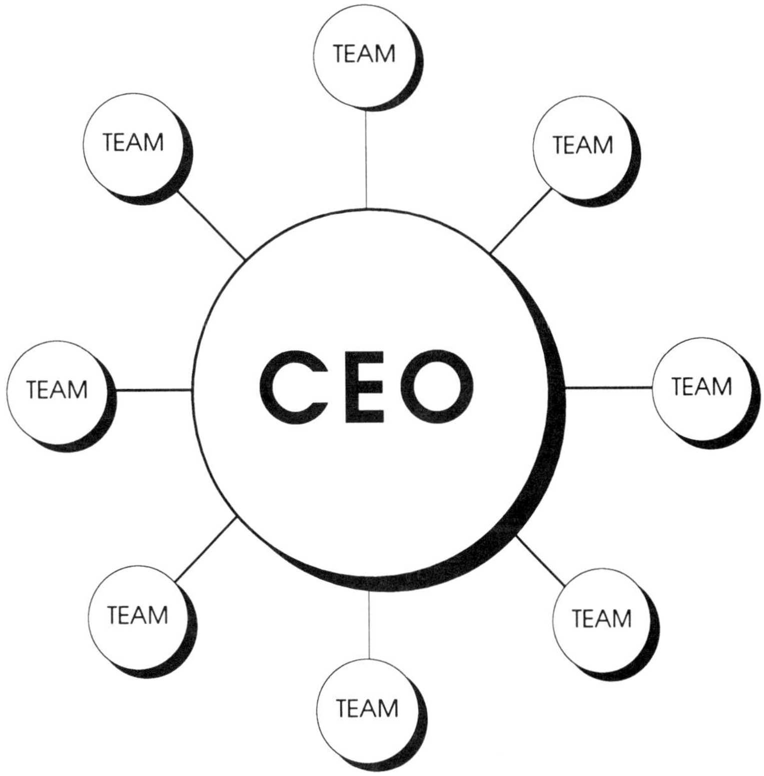

effort. This approach offers the dynamic advantage of adaptability and flexibility. From a performance management perspective, it suggests that both group and individual contributions will need to be tracked. It also suggests a multi-skilled team approach.

Some health care organizations, particularly those who have streamlined, have also adopted the cross-training approach. They often use a matrix organizational structure with functions being handled by several staff pulled from several departments. Supervisors thus may have staff reporting to them for certain assignments and reporting to others for other assignments. In this case, performance plans and reviews must be done in a group management context.

In smaller medical practices, a "family" or community style of management can be very conducive to a group or team. This size of practice also can find it advantageous to celebrate together when organizational goals are achieved.

Job analysis and job description

Once the plans and the organizational structure are in place, the human resource team must carefully analyze the critical factors of each job — another major objective of the performance management system. If the jobs presently exist in the organization, the analyst needs to interview jobholders and supervisors to ensure there is current information on such items as supervision received and exercised, equipment used, working conditions, responsibilities, duties, accountabilities and qualifications. (See Figure 3.4 on page 44.)

If the position does not currently exist in the organization, the job analyst must interview others in organizations that have this function. Sometimes this will mean crossing over into other industries. For example, if the clinic wants to add the position of client service representative, the job analyst may need to interview not only other clinics and hospitals, but also other service industries such as durable medical equipment vendors and insurance companies.

Out of this data should come updated job descriptions that will serve as the framework for identifying specific behavioral duty statements and expected outcomes. This becomes a critical document throughout the entire human resource process — from recruiting to orientation to performance planning and evaluation. (See Figure 3.5 on page 46.)[3]

Performance standards

The next objective is ensuring that job descriptions are complemented by performance standards that clearly spell out the yardsticks of success. For example, a job duty statement from the job description that specifies "Examine patients" will have a related performance standard that states "Examine 10-12 patients per day, on schedule."

The job duty "greet patients" will be matched with the standard "Greet each patient with a smile. Refer to them by name. Tell them how long they will have to wait. Offer them a magazine and coffee."

The standards must be built on quantity, quality, cost and timeliness factors. The point: It must be perfectly clear what kind and level of performance is expected.

Chapter Five , "Developing a performance management system," provides examples on how to develop such standards.

Preparing the organization

As the medical practice develops its philosophy on performance management, its strategic plan and organizational chart and the steps toward a new performance management process, it should be sharing these steps with supervisors in terms of contemplated changes. These discussions, which over time should involve more and more employees, begin the development and implementation phases, an important objective of the system.

That is, input from as many sources as possible is critical from step one when a new system is being developed. As supervisors and staff have an opportunity to shape the system, they will also be determining how to implement it effectively and how to orient users. An excellent way to

Figure 3.4

Sample job analysis tool

Job Analysis Questionnaire

I. GENERAL DATA

1. Department ______________________ Date ______________________
2. Name of Incumbent ______________________ Data Obtained from ______________________
3. Position Title ______________________

II. ORGANIZATION RELATIONSHIPS

4. Employees supervised:

	Number	Title
a)		
b)		
c)		
d)		
e)		
f)		
g)		
h)		
i)		

5. Total number supervised ______________________
6. Supervision received ______________________
7. Equipment operated ______________________
8. Working conditions: ______________________
9. Organization of department (draw an organization chart for incumbent's part of the organization).

Department title ______________________

III. DUTIES OF THE POSITION

10. a) ______________________

b) ______________________

c) ______________________

d) ______________________

e) ______________________

f) ______________________

g) ______________________

h) ______________________

i) ______________________

j) ______________________

11. Major outputs of unit supervised: ______________________________

____

____

____

____

____

IV. QUALIFICATIONS REQUIRED BY POSITION

12. Education required: ______________________________

____

____

____

____

____

13. Experience required: ______________________________

____

____

____

____

____

14. Special requirements (specify): ______________________________

____

____

____

____

____

15. License requirements: ______________________________

____

____

____

____

____

16. Required knowledge, skills and abilities: ______________________________

____

____

____

____

____

____

Prepared by Date

Source: Medical Group Management Association, Denver, Colo.

Figure 3.5

Sample job description tool

Position description

Position title ______________________________

General statement of duties ______________________________

____

Supervision received ______________________________

____

Supervision exercised ______________________________

____

Essential functions (Responsibility statements with related duties and procedures) ______________

____

____

____

Guidelines statement (This description of responsibilities is intended to provide only basic guidelines for meeting each responsibility. Additional responsibilities may be added, as appropriate.) ________

____

____

____

Education ______________________________

____

Experience ______________________________

____

Special requirements ______________________________

____

Knowledge ______________________________

____

Skills ______________________________

____

____

Abilities ______________________________

____

____

Working conditions ______________________________

____

____

____

Equipment operated ______________________________

____

____

involve staff in such planning is to establish a Performance Focus task force. This group should be representative of all functions in the medical practice and be expected to cross-fertilize ideas.

This implementation phase also includes a focus on training. Managers must give careful consideration to how the new performance management system will be communicated to supervisors and employees.

Part of this can be handled by traditional communication modes, such as new supervisor and employee performance handbooks, or articles in the organization's newsletter and presentations by management to the entire staff. Supplies of the new forms should be available to everyone to review and opportunities for questions should be provided. Information on when and how the system will start must be shared.

Other methods include bringing in an outside consultant to help facilitate skill-building workshops such as having supervisors rehearse performance feedback sessions. Videos also can be used to show the correct ways to use the tools and the process.

One of the best ways to get the implementation is to use the Performance Focus task force as the communicators and the trainers. Those staff members who helped design the system are the best advocates and experts.

Training for supervisors should be scheduled and completed within a certain timeframe. And this training should be available whenever a new supervisor is appointed and a review session scheduled each year.

Performance plans

After everyone is up to speed on the system, the next step is for each supervisor to sit down with each employee and negotiate a performance plan. Depending on the format of the system chosen (Chapter Five provides several samples), this discussion may focus primarily on such performance factors as quantity and quality, using some general descriptors or very specific behavioral language. Or the supervisor and employee may establish some objectives with quantitative measures.

Regardless of the format used, the intent of this session is to link the medical practice's objectives with the individual's job performance and development. This type of planning helps the employee to understand what the organization wants to achieve and to see how important his or her contribution is to the whole.

The main purpose for this upfront planning is communication — agreeing on performance expectations at the beginning so the employee will have a clear path to follow.

Once the system is in place, such performance planning is done regularly with every new employee and every time an employee assumes a new position. Then at the end of every year, the results of the plan are reviewed and a new plan for the next year is developed.

Monitoring

Once the plan is in place, the supervisor and employee track progress. This tracking can be tied to specific monthly performance indicators such as budget reports, number of clients seen or number of customer complaints.

It also can be tied to critical incidents, such as significant occurrences that are examples of successful behavior or inappropriate behavior. Supervisors, as part of their ongoing observation and feedback, should be constantly watching for these benchmarks of behavior and documenting them immediately. These documents are then shared with the employee as a means of reinforcing what works or doesn't work.

Feedback is the key to effective monitoring. Employees need to know if they are on target. Hopefully the performance goals and standards are so specific that they will be able to monitor success themselves. In any case, they will appreciate knowing that their supervisors are paying attention and are taking the time to communicate their observations.

Evaluation

Monitoring is a form of evaluation, thus ideally evaluation is occurring constantly. To ensure information is consolidated frequently, it is useful for the supervisor to meet often with the employee to check, "How's it going?," generally, and specifically, "How is XYZ coming along?"

These sessions could be as often informally as once a day for a new employee, or weekly or monthly for employees with more experience. At a minimum, quarterly reviews are recommended. Some medical practices have comprehensive reviews every six months; others do this once a year. There should always be a formal opportunity for the employee to know, "How am I doing?" In all cases, evaluation in some form should be ongoing and should be the responsibility of both the supervisor and employee.

Performance problems

No supervisor, no organization can afford not to identify and/or not deal with the fact that a performer is having a problem. The results of ignorance of such situations can range from a minor annoyance to a maximum explosion with severe personnel and legal consequences.

Thus, one of the objectives of a performance management process is to ensure that it includes mechanisms for identifying, analyzing and dealing with performance problems. One of these mechanisms is upfront prevention through careful selection and orientation of employees, followed by a negotiated performance plan. Hopefully, these steps will ensure that the employee is qualified to perform the job and can meet the expectations.

The second mechanism is the ongoing monitoring and evaluation. As the supervisor observes the employee, any deviation from the performance plan should be evident ... particularly when a pattern of repeated mistakes occurs.

As discussed more thoroughly in a later chapter, such incidents must be dealt with immediately and directly. With thoughtful problem-solving and assistance, the majority should have successful results.

Rewards

Another objective of a performance management system is to ensure that appropriate performance is rewarded and recognized appropriately. As explained in Chapter Ten, such compensation typically involves monetary rewards, provided in a variety of ways and at a variety of times, and cashless compensation.

Cashless compensation or "psychic pay" should be provided consistently by positive feedback. It also should be provided via formal recognition systems (mentions in the organizational newsletter and at "awards" occasions). Rewards also should come in the form of job enrichment; more responsibility, new challenges. Spontaneously celebrating success (individual and team) is an excellent way to give feedback and reinforce outstanding performance.

> "One of our objectives is to have the performance process help the employee to take responsibility for the job — rather than just for doing a task. We hope they will take ownership for doing the job as they see it should be done. Then their commitment will be stronger and there is more accomplishment. When they are empowered, they have a sense of ownership and the job takes on a new perspective. They are not just following the job description."
>
> *(MGMA member, medium-size clinic)*

Updating

A key objective of a performance management process is that it is maintained and updated consistently. Times, values, people, organizations and performance objectives will change. New methods and tools should be developed. Bugs will be found in the current system and should be identified and improved upon.

For all these reasons, the system's managers should have a built-in schedule for reviewing it. Often an outside consultant can provide thoughts on new ways of doing things. Frequently health care conventions and publications will alert medical practices to new approaches.

But supervisors and employees are the best insurance against system decay and obsolescence. If the process isn't working, or if they are aware of better ways, they should let the medical practice managers know. These managers must be open to revising the system.

Human resource experts recommend that job descriptions be reviewed annually for major changes and that each job be re-analyzed at least every two years. And, at least once every three years, the entire process should be reviewed to make sure it's the best it can be.

Human resources functions

As this discussion of the objectives of a performance management process confirms, every human resource function has a performance component. (See Figure 3.6) The process links organizational goals with personnel goals related to recruiting/selection, orientation/training, personnel movement and compensation and serves as the thread that weaves all these functions together.[4]

Figure 3.6

Human resource wheel

The performance management process is the center of the human resource wheel of functions: selection, orientation/training, personnel movement, compensation.

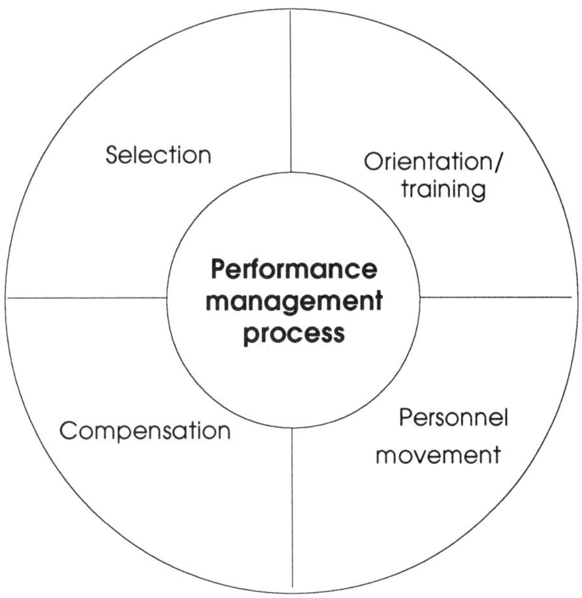

Source: The Group Practice Personnel Policies Manual, Medical Group Management Association.

Selection

Selection begins with human resource forecasting that is based on the medical practice's strategic performance plan. This forecasting aims to determine what personnel the organization will need to maintain its growth and exploit future opportunities.

These forecasters try to predict the number, type and quality of employees needed in the future; specify the range of responsibilities that will have to be met; establish the skills and knowledge needed; and document these responsibilities and qualifications in job descriptions.

Once this is done, the human resource professional can recruit the kind of qualified employees the organization needs, using the job description as the means for building a profile of the "best performer." Supervisors then can use this template when interviewing job applicants and will have a far better chance of selecting the person with the most potential for success. Applicants also will have a much better chance of making a wise decision about whether or not to accept a job offer, if performance standards are made clear during the process.

Orientation and training

Once a new employee is on board, the section in the employee handbook about the performance management process can be used to introduce the person to the "way we do it here." The process should be carefully explained and the tools used should be shared.

As the supervisor orients the employee to the position and its responsibilities, the job description and related performance standards will direct the discussions toward specific expectations. One of these discussions should result in a performance plan for the new employee, usually for a specific introductory period.

The expectations for this time period should be clear and should not only give the employee a real "taste test" of the job, but also should be structured to allow the person to make small win-win steps toward success. Usually performance expectations are based on minimum performance standards for this brief time. After that, a longer-range plan is put into effect.

Personnel movement

Most medical practices try to offer some opportunities for employee movement within the organization although this is dependent on the size of the group. This usually means promotion. Most individuals like to develop new skills to advance and to take on new challenges and responsibilities. This also might mean a lateral transfer. Occasionally it may mean a demotion or a layoff. Hopefully it rarely means termination.

Once again, job descriptions, performance standards and performance plans play a major part in such decisions. An individual's performance track record will be reviewed when openings occur or when layoffs are considered.

Succession planning usually is built with the performance management process in mind. In this case, the medical practice plans ahead in terms of filling position slots over time, such as who will be groomed for the next medical director opening, or how fast to move Mary up the career ladder. Such decisions on who gets ahead are based on how closely and quickly individuals show that they have the “right stuff” as evaluated by the performance process.

Terminations, of course, must have as their foundation a very solid and documented performance management process. The decision to fire an employee has momentous impacts on the organization, the supervisor and the employee. Such decisions must be made slowly and carefully after taking many steps to ensure it is the only answer.

Termination also may occur through no fault of the employee. A medical practice may need to downsize and lay off employees. Or it may choose to restructure and not be able to appropriately retrain all employees. In these cases, the decisions also must be based on legitimate performance and business necessity criteria.

Compensation

Compensation administration is a combination of identifying what a job is worth to the organization (how it will help the medical practice achieve the performance it desires), what a job is worth externally (the competitive market rate) and how the actual jobholder performs that brings value to the organization.

Critical steps that tie compensation administration and performance management relate to how the medical practice decides to handle pay increases. For example:

- Are these made on the basis of tenure and seniority? (Is the organization's performance improved because of employee longevity?)
- Are they made on the basis of merit? (The individual has performed in a meritorious fashion.)
- Is pay directly tied to performance? (Is there a reward if an individual achieves a certain goal within a certain time?)

- Does the organization wish to reward achievement after the fact (merit raises) or inspire future performance through incentives?

- Does the organization have a comprehensive menu of cashless compensation options that can be used with the discretion of the supervisor?

Whatever the decisions, employees and supervisors must understand how compensation correlates with performance. They will remember the performance-reward cycle; that is, "I perform, you reward ... then I will perform again." This is the implicit contract between employer and employee.

Summing up

Performance management is useful to organizations and employees in many ways. The key focus is the important part it plays in conjunction with strategic planning and human resource planning. It is an integral part in the successful functioning of any business, but especially in service businesses like the health care field.

Organizational and personal development are best served when reasonably high performance goals are set and achieved. A properly developed and executed performance management process is a means for both setting and recognizing the achievement of goals. It promotes maximum results from the wise investment of human resources.

Footnotes

[1]*James A. F. Stoner, Charles Wankel.* Management. *Englewood Cliffs, N.J.: Prentice-Hall, 1986, p. 53.*

[2]*Courtney Price, Alys Novak.* Health Care Innovation and Venture Trends. *Albany, N.Y.: Delmar Publishing Co., 1992, p. 209.*

[3]*Courtney Price.* The Group Practice Job Description Handbook. *Denver, Colo.: Medical Group Management Association, 1991.*

[4]*Courtney Price.* The Group Practice Personnel Policies Manual. *Denver, Colo.: Medical Group Management Association, 1991.*

Supervisory responsibilities for managing performance

Chapter Four

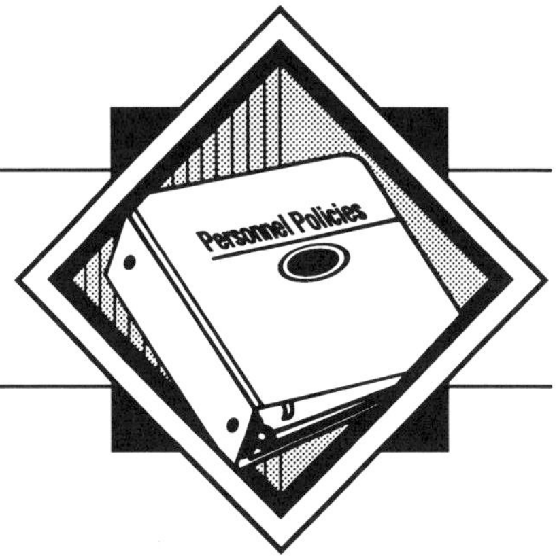

Recently a medical practice manager promoted a very competent lab technician to the position of supervisor of the department. The woman's technical expertise was top-notch and she had been with the organization for three years. The previous supervisor, who had retired, had often pointed out her superior performance to others in the department. And, she had many friends in the department. The manager was very pleased that the perfect person was available — until he began to hear grumbles from the department staff and from other staff who used the laboratory. There were constant reports of conflicts with the supervisor, with late reports, missing specimens. The manager mentioned his dilemma one day to a colleague, who asked: "Has this person ever supervised before?" Upon hearing that she had not, the colleague said: "This person does not know what a supervisor's job is. You should consider sending her to a supervisory training course."

To repeat a point: management is performance management. Management is all about getting work done through others. More specifically, effective supervision involves setting success standards and providing the support necessary to ensure success.

In short, supervisors have the prime responsibility for the performance management system. They can be most effective in doing this by integrating the concepts of performance management into their everyday supervisory tasks of planning, organizing, leading and controlling.

Supervisors also are the prime beneficiaries of an effective performance management system. A uniform framework for performance management helps them set specific, job-related performance expectations with employees, give feedback on a regular basis as year-long coaches and take the gloom and doom out of the year-end performance evaluation session.

First-line responsibility

Supervisors have a unique role in the performance management system, and in management in general. Of all the managers in a medical practice, including the CEO, the senior managers, the middle managers, the practitioners — first-line supervisors are the most important in terms of getting the work done.[1]

They are the ones who:

- work the closest with the work units/teams;
- personally deal with employees on a regular basis;
- have the best opportunity to observe performance and to correct/praise it immediately; and
- see patterns developing over time in terms of performance improvement or performance deviation.

They should be the ones who:

- provide assistance and guidance;
- serve as teachers, coaches, cheerleaders; and
- explain what the game is, how to win it, how it will be scored and when.

They are not only on the line to bring home the trophy to the owners of the team, but also they are the bottom line in terms of ensuring that organizational goals are achieved. (See Figure 4.1)

Figure 4.1

Supervisors on the line

Supervisors are the key to getting the work done through people for these reasons:

- They work closely with employees.
- They deal with employees one on one.
- They observe performance and praise/correct it.
- They see patterns of improvement/ deviation.
- They teach, coach, counsel, reward.

Supervisory perspective

Often an individual is promoted from the work unit to become its supervisor. This makes sense since he/she has had the opportunity to learn about the jobs and the team members by being part of the group and its activities.

However, when this "suddenly you are a supervisor" move occurs, new supervisors need to readjust their attention from just focusing on doing the work, to helping others do the work. This means acquiring a new set of skills.

It also means gaining a new perspective about what's important. Now is the time for supervisors to:

- get in tune with the big picture — the goals of the entire organization, not just those of an individual performer or those of the unit;
- understand strategic objectives for long-term success;
- recognize the importance of interdepartmental cooperation;
- see their team as one part of a much bigger team with a common mission and success target; and
- understand their new role and coach and facilitator.

Like any employee, they must work with their managers to gain this new perspective and new skills. And they must negotiate a performance plan so they, too, understand their performance expectations.

New supervisor challenges

Whether the new supervisor is a physician or a nurse or a lab technician or a medical records clerk, it cannot be assumed that just because the person is technically competent, he or she will be competent as a supervisor. Two sins often occur when individuals are promoted to a supervisory position. The employees are not:

- assessed to confirm they have an interest in or aptitude for supervision; or

- given supervisory training and management support.

First, medical practices should arrange for supervisory assessment. The fact is that some individuals are better suited to be individual performers than to be supervisors of others. It is very costly in terms of time and effort to promote a person with a high probability of failure in this vital position. Therefore, it is very worthwhile having the human resource specialist conduct a supervisory aptitude assessment or send the person to a counselor who specializes in career assessments.

It is also valuable to invest in supervisory training. Even if a person has performed satisfactorily before as a supervisor, it will be important to provide education on "how we do it here and now." If the medical practice does not have on-site training available, the human resource professional can guide the new supervisor to the many courses offered. There are also many good books available for learning and polishing supervisory skills, as noted in the Additional Resources section.

In addition, assigning a mentor to the new supervisor is useful. This usually is not the supervisor's manager. Other senior employees can better serve as the new supervisor's coach.

In addition to the need for training, new supervisors also often need help facing a common dilemma. If they are promoted out of the unit they will be supervising, they have gotten used to being a "pal" to the other team members. All of a sudden, they must be setting expectations and evaluating the performance of their buddies. This typically causes great discomfort for the supervisor and sometimes for the team.

Through training and with management's help, the new supervisor can face this challenge with honesty and openness. Indeed, this is an excellent opportunity to reinforce the value of the performance management process. The supervisor can very effectively use this framework to establish new relationships with team members that are objective and job related. This takes much of the personal discomfort out of the interactions.

Once supervisors see how this approach helps to achieve the unit's performance goals and to guide their everyday relations with employees, they will become the strongest supporters of the process. This support, of course, is contingent on top management's providing an effective process and the help supervisors need — and giving them time to supervise by reducing their "doing" tasks.

Planning

The first skill supervisors must utilize to ensure effective team performance is planning. Planning is defined as determining what should be done and why, and then figuring out the logistics — how, when, where, who.[2]

There are several different kinds of planning:

- **Strategic long-range planning**. This typically is done by the top managers with supervisory input;

- **Annual operational plans**. Supervisors usually become more involved in developing these plans by working with their managers to establish goals and objectives for their departments;

- **Action work plans**. These plans for the unit/team are very much the supervisor's responsibility. Once the work plan is established, supervisors develop plans to help the team accomplish its tasks. (See Figure 4.2) These steps include:

  - acquire needed resources;
  - develop a budget;
  - assign work;
  - schedule work;
  - establish checkpoints and deadlines;
  - develop an implementation strategy;
  - consider any constraints;
  - clarify performance expectations and standards; and
  - determine how results will be evaluated.

Figure 4.2

Supervisory planning tasks

Supervisors plan what to do, and how, when, where, who, including planning related to:

- ✔ resources;
- ✔ budgets;
- ✔ assignments;
- ✔ schedules;
- ✔ timelines;
- ✔ implementation;
- ✔ contingencies;
- ✔ expectations; and
- ✔ evaluation.

In effect, this work planning is unit performance planning. It then serves as the basis for developing performance plans for each employee.

Some medical practices do not have a long-range strategic plan nor an annual organizational plan. In this case, it is still appropriate for supervisors to do action work plans on an annual basis. Or, they can develop project plans rather than a year-long master plan.

The same approach is used on a smaller scale. The supervisor will have to consider the need for personnel, information, equipment, supplies, as well as the need to schedule activities and to define results.

Project planning is often a great opportunity for medical practice supervisors in terms of learning how to:

- set goals with team members;
- delegate responsibilities;
- problem-solve together; and
- develop the skills of others.

One great developmental exercise is the "what if" game. This involves contingency planning. What if the project leader must take a leave of absence; what if the vendor doesn't get the supplies here on time; what if there is a power outage? By establishing a game plan that includes fallback "Plan B," the project team and supervisor have some performance insurance.

When the annual team planning is complete, the supervisor meets with each employee to develop the personalized performance plan (sample forms shown in Chapter Five). This involves more than simply instructing an employee on assigned tasks. To ensure that employees can perform at their best, a more appropriate approach includes several steps. (See Figure 4.3) These include:

- clarifying the purposes of the assignment;
- specifying the nature of the assignment;
- listening to the employee's views; he or she may have ideas that are better than the supervisor's;

Figure 4.3

Planning checklist

Supervisors should be able to answer "Yes" to these questions.

✔ Have I clarified the purpose of the assignment?

✔ Have I specified the nature of the assignment?

✔ Have I listened to the employee's views?

✔ Have I shared relevant knowledge?

✔ Have I made sure the employee can do the task?

✔ Have I made sure resources are available?

✔ Have I confirmed that rewards are available?

✔ Have I discussed performance checkpoints?

✔ Have I stressed the importance of two-way feedback?

✔ Have I specified performance review times?

- sharing relevant knowledge in a coaching style;
- making sure the employee has the ability, skills and motivation to do the task;
- verifying that the resources necessary to do the task are available, including people, equipment, funds, authority;
- confirming that the pay, incentives and other benefits make it worthwhile for the employee to try hard;
- discussing how the supervisor will observe performance;
- agreeing on how and when feedback will be shared, including encouraging the employee to take the initiative; and
- specifying when and how evaluations will occur.

As discussed more thoroughly in a later chapter, this performance communication model is similar to the "One-Minute Manager" approach developed by Blanchard and Johnson. Blanchard says, "The idea is simple. Set goals with subordinates. Observe and monitor their performance. Give them positive feedback when they do something right, and reprimand them when they do something wrong."[3]

Not only does this approach represent common sense, it also is a powerful supervisory practice that keeps everyone on target.

Organizing

Another key skill for supervisors is organizing. Organizing is defined as: setting up an administrative structure for getting things done. This involves arranging workers into a productive unit. This results in synergy — the whole is greater than the sum of the parts. This includes improving the:

- organizational structure of the unit;
- reporting relationships;

- coordination; and
- efficient use of resources.

After the work unit's goals have been identified, it is critical to analyze the operations performed in the unit. One way to do this is to draw a flow chart of the tasks that must be accomplished and indicate the flow of information necessary to meet these goals.

Next, study the work unit's organization chart to get answers to these questions:

- Are there lead workers/team leaders who share supervisory responsibilities?
- Who reports to whom and what are these responsibilities?
- Does the chart reveal any duplication of effort?
- Are any employees performing functions not directly related to the accomplishment of unit goals?
- Do employees lack the skills needed to attain goals?
- Are there too many or too few individuals available to accomplish the work load for any step of the process?

If there are any questions about the effectiveness of the present structure, the supervisor should discuss it with his or her manager. Together they can come up with a more efficient approach. For example, they may consider a multi-skilled team approach that forms into different configurations based on the project.

The supervisor will also want to look at the numbers of employees supervised. If the number is more than seven, it is likely that the supervisor will not be able to give each employee the kind of performance coaching they deserve. In this case, delegating coaching/mentoring responsibilities to team leaders makes sense.

In terms of coordination, supervisors play a key role in ensuring that every employee understands each other's responsibilities and how they impact each other's performance. Horizontal communication should be stressed — what each person is doing and why, and how we can help

> "We hope that supervisors will see that it's a whole lot easier when employees are empowered. The initial fears about empowerment were that there would be anarchy. That is not happening. The quality movement has attached a lot of hugs and kisses to the supervisor-employee relationships. It isn't saying that. It means still doing the job in a quality manner and being accountable for results — and doing this with a positive approach. Right now there is a lot of flip-flopping. Supervisors are going back and forth between macho management/tough guy to buddy-buddy/nice guy. Neither works. Partners in performance works."
>
> *(MGMA member, medium-sized clinic)*

each other. The supervisor is also responsible for external communication — coordinating information and efforts with other units.

In addition, the supervisor should check to see if performance could be improved by reorganizing work flow, space or information flow. Perhaps computers could be used more efficiently. Perhaps medical records could be handled differently as they move through the process from admissions to service to charting to billing.

Once again, employees can provide valuable input about ways to organize that will improve performance. One major payoff: More effective organization usually leads to more effective time management.

Leading

Over time leadership has been defined in a variety of ways ... as authority, as power, as charisma. Today the standard definition of leadership skills is the ability to be a visionary planner and to empower others.

As stated by Oakley and Krug, "Enlightened leaders are clear about the importance of a mission that incorporates a vision of what the organization stands for or strives to create that is inspiring and elevating to the team."[4]

This very contemporary definition reinforces the premise that no organization, no medical practice will survive if its leaders cannot envision future success and plan the performance steps necessary to get there. And since no one person can make an organization successful, it's necessary to entrust workers with much more responsibility than ever before — in the name of achieving precise performance objectives together.

As noted previously, supervisors should be part of the strategic planning, which includes envisioning a desired future. They then can reinforce this vision everyday with the unit/team and with the individual performer. Example: Many medical practices today have a vision of being recognized as providing quality service to patients. Supervisors can both talk the talk about quality and walk this talk through their role modeling of what quality means for the unit and how to achieve it.

Figure 4.4

Motivation tips

Employees are motivated by:

- clear expectations;
- managing their performance;
- frequent feedback;
- supervisor support;
- achieving their goals and objectives; and
- appropriate rewards.

Supervisors also need to role model other behaviors that are characteristic of leaders, including being:

- futuristic;
- energetic;
- enthusiastic;
- ethical; and
- optimistic.

Supervisors who come in everyday with high energy and high spirits, with high ethical standards and a high level of optimism and a vision of the future will provide the motivating conditions that employees need to perform successfully. Even though supervisors cannot motivate workers since motivation occurs within an individual, they do play a major role in providing many of the rewards that individuals seek and in eliminating many of the barriers to performance that employees encounter. (See Figure 4.4)

For example, employees are motivated to perform effectively when they:

- know what is expected of them;
- manage their performance;
- receive feedback on and reinforcement of their performance;
- can achieve their own goals and objectives;
- can count on supervisors to remove such barriers to motivation as inappropriate compensation, inadequate working conditions and insufficient resources; and
- feel that their supervisors try hard to:
    - match their responsibilities with their abilities;
    - provide opportunities for advancement;
    - support efforts for personal growth; and
    - help them acquire a sense of achievement.

Empowerment can be as simple as having workers who previously prepared reports for their supervisors' signature now be authorized to sign themselves ... and to be held accountable for those reports. It also can mean something more sophisticated; i.e., loosening managerial controls to give workers increased responsibilities for managing their own work. As noted previously, self-managing teams are an example of empowerment that is very motivating.

A vital key to leadership and to motivation is for supervisors to understand that each individual usually requires a different style of leadership. For example, the work of Blanchard and Hershey on "situational leadership," is based on the premise that an individual needs to be supervised based on his or her ability and motivation.

For example, they recommend that the most effective leadership style to use with a employee assuming a new job is a "telling" style. The premise: this worker may be willing but is basically ignorant about what to do and/or how to do it here. Thus, it is the supervisor's responsibility to tell him or her about the job by showing how to do it.

Once the worker has demonstrated some ability, the supervisor then can use a "selling" style by doing it together with the employee. This stage also involves reinforcing (selling) the successful way of doing it and increases motivation.

After the worker has demonstrated competence, the supervisor steps to the sidelines and uses a "coaching" style. Now the worker does it himself or herself and the supervisor provides guidance. The coaching continues over time to ensure the expected level of performance continues. This is especially important to maintain motivation.

In some cases, upon repeated demonstrations of successful performance, the supervisor can move to a "delegating" style — "It's all yours, go for it!" In the past, this often meant relinquishing all responsibility for the task and a "whatever works" attitude. Today, empowerment means accountability for the individual and team — and for the supervisor/coach, who is charged with providing the standards and support necessary for quality and success, even in the delegation stage.[5]

Other skills of leadership include:

- oral and written communication;
- envisioning the future clearly and concisely;

- problem identification and solving;
- decision making; and
- group dynamics.

> “Our goals: To have supervisors not worry about friendships when evaluating employees. They would do honest appraisals. They would do planning upfront. They would not be encumbered by the buddy system.”
>
> *(MGMA member, medium-sized medical practice)*

There are many courses available to help new supervisors gain these skills. The important point to emphasize when considering such learning is: Leaders are the servants of the group. No one can be a leader if no one follows him or her. A group of workers must feel that their leader, their supervisor, is capable of leading the group to success. They expect supervisors to be:

- articulate in communicating to them and to others about their needs and successes;
- proficient in working with the group to solve problems and to reach decisions; and
- able to “conduct the group” like an orchestra so their performance hits the right note.

Controlling

From a supervisory point of view, the word “control” is not defined in the punitive or restrictive or possessive sense. Rather, control is defined as monitoring and correcting.

A good analogy of such control is situational leadership as demonstrated by a mother teaching her child to walk across the street safely. When the little girl is just starting to walk, the mother tells the child that she is too little to do this herself. So she picks her up and carries her across the street. Then as the child gains walking ability, the mother takes her by the hand and they walk together across the street. Next, the child goes across the street herself while mother stands on the curb and calls out correcting comments. When the child has shown she can successfully do this and is willing to do it correctly, mother stays in the house and the child is on her own.

Another way of defining control is delegation. As workers gain more skill and interest, more is delegated to them. Shame on the supervisor who keeps control of everything. Not only cannot one person do everything, but no one else is learning or is motivated by such action.

Delegation, of course, is a skill in itself. It means looking at each task and each decision and determining if the supervisor must retain and perform it, or it can be shared with workers or can be delegated to employees. The "musts" that the supervisor should keep should be few and based on key result accountabilities. Other tasks should be delegated as appropriate. "Appropriate" in this case means these things:

- using employees' strengths when delegating. Reviewing their performance evaluations will help in this process. Also look at areas needing improvement to check if certain tasks could be used as development opportunities; and

- determining the amount of delegation ranging from:

  - proceed without approval;
  - proceed, but inform supervisor of actions; and
  - obtain approval before proceeding.

To start the delegation off successfully, it is necessary to identify:

- when the task is to be completed;

- where it is to be performed;

- how it should be accomplished;

- when and why feedback will be given; and

- when interim and final progress reports are required.

This is a performance plan that demonstrates control in its best form; i.e., setting expectations, monitoring, correcting.

The most important step of delegation, especially in the beginning, is checking employees' progress. Be sure to expect and review progress reports quickly and carefully, do occasional spot checks and set aside time to discuss progress and problems. Make sure performance is successful by controlling/monitoring its path all the way to a productive conclusion.

Summing up

"We would like supervisors to be able to decatastrophsize — to not make a big deal out of small things. Supervisors get caught up in focusing on the things that are not quite right, that they don't see what's wonderful. Probably that's because the medical world focuses on what's wrong ... we are always looking for the problem. Supervisors should accentuate the positive. Everyone needs champions.

"Also in terms of conditioning, along the way supervisors should help make employees understand the responsibility that management has. The supervisor has to answer for results. So supervisors need the input and participation of employees. Supervision is all about leadership, and with every leadership role is an obligation to say when something is wrong."

(MGMA member, small, rural medical practice)

Successful performance for a supervisor means acting like a leader:

- Create and express the vision;
- Demonstrate commitment;
- Take responsibility for how well employees perform and improve;
- Pay attention to workers' needs and wants;
- Allow people to have spirit;
- Measure progress by noting how often everyone hits the success target;
- Act as a role model; and
- Be accountable to and for the work unit. Their performance depends on the supervisor's performance.

Russell Coile Jr., notes in *The New Medicine* that "Reduction of the middle ranks (of management) may actually increase administrative opportunities for front-line supervisors as part of the 'work site democracy' moment to decentralize authority and distribute it to the operating units."[6]

As this occurs, Peter Senge says, "The leader's task is designing the learning processes whereby people throughout the organization can deal productively with the critical issues they face, and develop their mastery in the learning disciplines. This is new work for most experienced managers, many of whom rose to the top because of their decision-making and problem-solving skills, not their skills in mentoring, coaching and helping others learn."[7]

The key then is coaching — the process of guided change in which interactive communication is used to gain the employee's support for new direction and changes. It provides an opportunity for the leader to act out and communicate organizational values, to confront specific situations where there is an opportunity for learning and to take immediate and full advantage of development opportunities as they occur.[8]

As Leland Kaiser, the health care futurist states, "As the health care organization grows more ephemeral, management will become an increasingly subtle art. Visionary skills are essential in a dynamic, rapidly changing society where the past is no longer a guide for the future."[9]

Footnotes

[1]*Richard Plunkett.* Supervision: The Direction of People at Work. *Dubuque, Iowa: Wm. C. Brown Co. Publishers, 1975.*

[2]*Lowell W. Hellervik, Brian L. Davis.* Improving Managerial Effectiveness. *Minneapolis, Minn.: Personnel Decisions, Inc., 1984.*

[3]*Kenneth Blanchard, Ph.D., Spencer Johnson, M.D.* The One-Minute Manager. *New York: Berkley Books, 1981.*

[4]*Ed Oakley, Doug Krug.* Enlightened Leadership. *Denver, Colo.: Stone Tree Publishing, 1992, p. 134.*

[5]*James A. F. Stoner, Charles Wankel.* Management. *Englewood Cliffs, N.J.: Prentice-Hall, Inc., 1986, P. 460.*

[6]*Russell C. Coile Jr.* The New Medicine: Reshaping Medical Practice and Health Care Management. *Rockville, M.D.: Aspen Publishers, 1990, p. 35.*

[7]*Peter M. Senge.* The Fifth Discipline: The Art and Practice of the Learning Organization. *New York: Doubleday, 1990, p. 345.*

[8]*Steven J. Stower, Ph.D., Matt M. Starcevich, Ph.D.* The Coach: Creating Partnerships for a Competitive Edge. *Salt Lake City, Utah: The Center for Management and Organization Effectiveness, 1987, p. 183.*

[9]*Leland R. Kaiser, Ph.D.* Role of Health Care Workers in the Future Delivery of Health Care. *Brighton, Colo.: Kaiser & Associates, 1991, p. 73.*

Developing a performance management system

Chapter Five

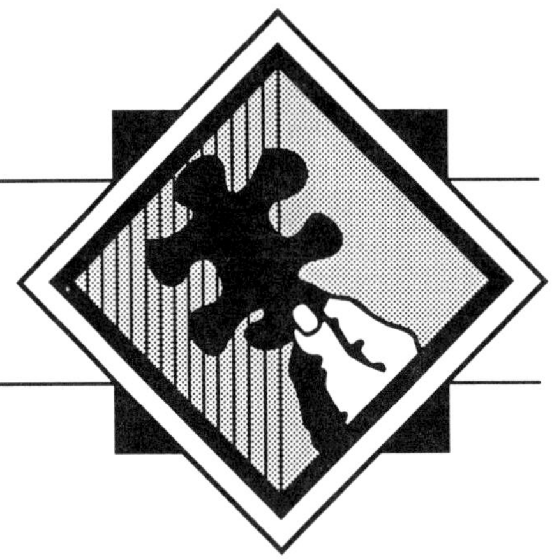

Figure 5.1

Performance management process flowchart

organization assessment
↓
policy decisions/ management input
↓
performance management process design
↓
design review
↓
pilot
↓
process finalization
↓
user orientation materials
↓
supervisory training materials
↓
dissemination/ communication

The management team of a small medical practice meets to discuss its performance evaluation system. Several managers have been reading a lot about the inadequacies of traditional evaluation approaches. They are also hearing rumbles of discontent from supervisors and employees about the "performance game." The forms currently used focus on personality traits rather than job-related behaviors, which embarrasses both the supervisors and the employees. The management team decides it's time to bring in a consultant who can suggest different approaches.

When starting on the development of a performance management system, there are several factors to consider, including (See Figure 5.1):

- history of the organization;
- organizational climate;
- policy decisions;

> “We revised our system three years ago. We tried to make it generic, but also have several specialized versions that are specific to task and department; e.g., clinical nursing, radiology, lab, receptionist. We have about a dozen nonexempt performance evaluation forms. The grading is 'meets standard, does not meet, exceeds.'”
>
> *(MGMA member, medium-sized group practice)*

- initial management input;
- performance process design;
- management and user review of design;
- pre-test;
- finalizing system;
- development of user orientation;
- development of supervisory training;
- preparation and dissemination of system procedures; and
- follow up, evaluation and revision.

Each of these steps takes careful consideration. However, the first is one of the most important. It is critical to assess the organization's history and then its current corporate culture in terms of its traditions, management style, size, life stage, economic health and strategic plan. Put more simply, it is important to determine what the physician/owners have done in the past, and what they are willing to do in the future.[1]

This analysis will help the designers develop the parameters for tailoring a performance management process for the medical practice. For example, if the medical practice is small (from one to 10 physicians), it will be best to design a system with few steps and components. If the practice is larger (over 20 physicians), with many types and levels of staff, a more elaborate system may be needed. If the practice is using TQM/CQI (which favors eliminating traditional performance evaluation), then it will need to be linked into the process in an innovative fashion.

The results of the analysis will help the medical practice to firm up its philosophy about performance. As discussed previously, before rolling out a new program or modifying an existing one, senior managers need to state their beliefs about performance management. This statement will be the driving force for:

- the system designers;
- the supervisors;
- the employees; and
- the human resource specialists.

This statement can be as simple as, "We have high standards of performance and expect employees to meet them. In turn, we believe in fair and consistent evaluation of performance to ensure employees' contributions are recognized and rewarded." Or, the statement could be more specific: "We believe in pay-for-performance. To accomplish this objective, we work with employees to set goals and we reward those who meet the goals."

The chosen statement should be communicated in a variety of ways: through supervisory training, employee publications and in particular, the medical practice's policy and procedures manual, and also in the employee handbook. This philosophy about performance will be especially important to share with new employees. It also will serve as a foundation for developing a legally defensible system.[2]

Policy decisions

Once the organizational objectives related to performance have been established, it is time to make a variety of decisions about the:

- type of tools (performance-standard method, criterion-based format, goal-setting device);
- emphasis on planning (specific performance goal-setting with each employee at the beginning of a performance period, or general planning tagged on to the end of a prior year's performance evaluation, as well as quarterly and/or midyear reviews);
- orientation of the new employee (a general introduction of the performance philosophy or a specific discussion of performance expectations based on the job description and a performance plan);

> "Under various categories we identify performance standards; e.g., quality (accuracy), quantity (timely), interpersonal skills, attendance, punctuality, safety, knowledge. We leave blank lines for the supervisor to add comments. We emphasize initiative and relationships with others."
>
> *(MGMA member, medium-sized clinic)*

- introduction of the new PMP to current staff (a general review or a specific training session);
- timing of the performance review (at the same time as the salary review or at a different time);
- focus of evaluation (the employee and/or the team);
- circle of evaluators (supervisor, self, peers, clients);
- involvement in system development (supervisors, employees, consultants, human resource professional, senior management, board); and
- compliance/appeal process (who reviews the reviewer; for example, supervisor's supervisor, human resource professional, CEO, and what steps should an employee take to grieve an evaluation?).

Employee involvement

The decision about employee involvement is a key one. A standard method is to assign the task of developing/revising the performance system to the human resource department in a larger group or to the manager with human resource responsibilities in a mid-size group and to the administrator or office manager in the smaller group, with review/approval by top management. However, as discussed previously, one of the recommended contemporary approaches to developing a performance management process is to involve multiple tiers in the larger organizations.

This approach fits today's emphasis on employee involvement and utilizes the classic premise of involving those who need to "buy into" the system in order to gain ownership in it. If this approach is used, the steps involved should include:

- Make a decision at the top management level to design/revise the current performance management process and develop a philosophy statement;
- Discuss the project with the remainder of the management team and obtain their initial input on needs, concerns and suggestions;

- Assign the project to the human resource professional or person responsible for these functions;

- Consider the use of a consultant to ensure a current and objective perspective, either to design the entire system or to provide guidance. The consultant also can conduct an organizational climate survey related to the performance environment (See Figure 5.2);

Figure 5.2

Organizational climate survey

Performance-related questions that can be used (and scaled from strongly agree to strongly disagree) in an organizational culture survey/climate analysis to get insights on employees' opinions about the environment in which they work include:

Scale

1 Not satisfied	2 Moderately satisfied	3 Satisfied	4 Very satisfied	5 Extremely satisfied

1. The organization helps me to progress in my career.
2. I am highly committed to the organization's mission.
3. Its goal-setting system is worthwhile.
4. High performance standards are set here.
5. Quality is as important as quantity here.
6. People here are reviewed on how well they perform.
7. People are paid appropriately for their position and performance.
8. People are recognized for doing a good job.
9. It's okay to fail when trying something new here.
10. The organization provides a good benefits package.
11. The organization is concerned about my personal career development.
12. My supervisor works with me to achieve realistic career objectives.
13. My supervisor helps me improve my performance.
14. My supervisor makes clear his/her priorities and expectations of me.
15. My supervisor is direct and honest with me.
16. My supervisor has realistic expectations of me.
17. My supervisor involves me in solving problems and making decisions.
18. My supervisor gives me timely feedback on how I'm doing.
19. My supervisor uses recognition and praise to reward me for excellent performance.

- Establish a Performance Focus task force to serve as advisors during the design and implementation stages. Invite representatives from key departments and include employees from every level from worker to supervisor to manager;

- Develop and administer an employee survey to gather opinions about the current process (See Figure 5.3); and

- Analyze this information and incorporate it into the design.

For smaller groups, the administrator or office manager can seek input from other staff and then proceed to develop the performance management plan.

Figure 5.3

Employee performance process survey

Questions that can be asked to get employee input on an organization's performance management process include:

1. How many times per year do you go through a formal review process with your supervisor?
2. How many times per year would you like to have a formal review with your supervisor?
3. Was your review process completed in a satisfactory period of time?
4. Would you rate the present process as a fair way to evaluate your job performance?
5. Does the present process help you improve your performance?
6. Does the process help you achieve your career goals?
7. Does the process help clarify your supervisor's job expectations?
8. If you were in charge of developing a new performance management process, what types of changes would you make?
9. What types of informal and formal feedback would help employees to improve their job performance?
10. Any other suggestions?
11. Are you an exempt or non-exempt employee?
12. Do you supervise any employees?

Performance evaluation tools

There are many different performance planning/evaluation formats. Each has its advantages and disadvantages. The major formats are described briefly. Then the three recommended for medical practices (performance standard, criterion, goal setting) are described in more detail and samples are provided. (See Figure 5.4 for a listing of format advantages and disadvantages.)[3]

Figure 5.4

Comparison of performance tools

There is no one "right" performance planning/evaluation tool. Each has advantages and disadvantages, as shown:

- **Essay**
  Review effectiveness dependent on evaluator's verbal skills
  Tendency to subjectivity
  Not recommended as sole method
  Useful as supplement to other methods

- **Critical incident**
  Review effectiveness dependent on evaluator's verbal skills
  Subject to evaluator's selection of incidents
  Perceived by employee as surveillance
  Useful focus on job behaviors
  Helpful documentation on problems — and successes

- **Peer/co-worker**
  Review effectiveness dependent on design of tool
  Confidentiality and cooperation critical
  Useful data source on ongoing performance
  Reinforcement of expected behaviors

- **Ranking focused on comparison among employees**
  No focus on individual performance
  Time-consuming design
  Little use for feedback

- **Behaviorally Anchored Rating Scale (BARS)**
  Objective, job-related criteria/standards
  Time-consuming to develop
  Useful as training/development tool

- **Management by objectives (MBO)**
  Tied to strategic plan
  Focused on mutual goal-setting/results
  Not applicable to all positions
  Time-consuming negotiations

Essay rating

Essay evaluation is a structured performance evaluation format that is minimally effective. Using this approach, appraisers comment on the employee's strengths, weaknesses, training needs, etc. While it can be a useful communication tool, such essays tend to be written subjectively, rather than focusing on specific job-related behaviors. Thus, the essay is no longer perceived as appropriate from a legal perspective, if it is the only method used.[4]

Also, not all supervisors can express themselves effectively in writing. One employee may receive an extensive, articulate essay rating, while another gets a terse, undescriptive rating. Although this approach is simple, it has little value in terms of improving performance and is fraught with subjectivity and potential legal hazards.

A valuable use of the essay approach is in combination with other approaches. That is, comments related to specific behaviors can be used to amplify other kinds of ratings.[4]

Critical incident rating

This approach is based upon an appraiser's written observation of an employee's performance throughout a designated time period. The supervisor maintains a log to record an employee's performance during work incidents that are considered critical, such as dealing with a patient. These sometimes are called significant occurrences. This listing of incidents/occurrences should be examples of both successful and unsatisfactory performance. (See Figure 5.5 on the following page.)

Since this approach is similar to the essay, it falls prey to the same problems in terms of the supervisor's verbal skills. However, it has the advantage of being more job related. Nevertheless, it can also be biased, by the incidents the supervisor chooses to record. It is a common fallacy to record only incidents that upset the supervisor. Supervisors forget to record incidents of exceptional performance because, in reality, they feel that type of behavior is expected.

Also, the approach, if done effectively, is very time consuming for the supervisor, requiring constant note taking and close observation. And, employees tend to consider

Figure 5.5

Critical incident form

This form can be used to note critical incidents/significant occurrences — both positive and negative — during the performance period. Both the supervisor and employee should discuss the incident, determine the appropriate action if correction is needed, and indicate this dis-cussion has taken place by signing the form.

Employee ______________________________

Title ______________________________

Supervisor ______________________________

Department ______________________________

Performance period: From __________ To __________
(Date)

Description ______________________________
____
____
____

Discussion action ______________________________
____
____
____
____
____

Signatures ______________________________
____
____

such constant observation as surveillance. Employees don't like having someone, particularly a supervisor, looking over their shoulders all day.

One positive use of this approach is to amplify specific job-related examples when using other formats. The approach is most useful, however, when dealing with performance problems. As explained in Chapter Eight, documentation of critical incidents is a vital step in developing a performance improvement plan and/or preparing to discipline or terminate an employee.[5]

Peer/co-worker review

The peer review method was originally designed for use in rating professional employees. It is frequently used in medical practices by physicians. In this process, a panel of colleagues confidentially rates the physician's performance. The main benefit of this system is that it allows for a credible rating by equals of a highly sophisticated workforce.

As discussed previously, peer/co-worker reviews are being redesigned by many health care organizations so they can be used by any work group to evaluate co-workers/peers in terms of such performance factors as patient relations, teamwork, quality. In time, co-worker reviews may become an integral part of the total performance plan/evaluation process and will be based upon performance factors and standards defined by the group. (See Figure 5.6 on the following page.)

Ranking methods

There are several performance evaluation tools that require the evaluator to compare employees. These tools include:

- paired comparison ranking, which involves comparing each employee in a job compared to all others in the group;
- alternation ranking, which involves evaluating all workers in a job group against a standard measure; and
- forced distribution ranking, which involves ranking employees on a universal measure according to a fixed proportion of the entire group.

The basic problem with the ranking approach is that it focuses on the group rather than the individual. It does not recognize that each person has a different level of experience in the job, has different strengths and weaknesses and may be on a different development path. Most important, ranking fails to identify individual differences in performance or inform the individual employee of how performance can be improved.[7]

Behaviorally anchored rating scale (BARS)

The BARS technique is a sophisticated measure of job performance that has a high degree of validity for any job; that is, it measures what it is supposed to measure. This

Figure 5.6

Co-worker performance evaluation form

This type of form can be used to gather employee performance information from co-workers.

Scale	1 Does not meet standard	2 Meets standard	3 Above standard	4 Exceeds standard

WORK QUANTITY: Volume of employee output including speed and consistency of work.
Standard: ____________________ Rating: ________
Comments: ____________________

WORK QUALITY: Extent to which work performance meets job requirements of accuracy and thoroughness.
Standard: ____________________ Rating: ________
Comments: ____________________

JOB KNOWLEDGE: Demonstration of skills or abilities necessary to perform job requirements.
Standard: ____________________ Rating: ________
Comments: ____________________

INITIATIVE: Degree of setting and attaining meaningful goals and taking action on own.
Standard: ____________________ Rating: ________
Comments: ____________________

DEPENDABILITY: Being punctual and following clinic policies/procedures.
Standard: ____________________ Rating: ________
Comments: ____________________

COMMUNICATION: Effectiveness of written and verbal reports.
Standard: ____________________ Rating: ________
Comments: ____________________

TEAMWORK: Skill and tact in influencing and giving/gaining cooperation.
Standard: ____________________ Rating: ________
Comments: ____________________

PATIENT RELATIONS: Display of respect, courtesy, friendliness, service with clients.
Standard: ____________________ Rating: ________
Comments: ____________________

OTHER COMMENTS: ____________________

Overall rating: ________

method uses an in-depth job analysis of work content and behavior for each job to be rated. Each job has a separate evaluation form that is specially tailored to a specific position.

BARS is an effective performance evaluation method because it produces highly objective, behavioral, job-related, quantitative rankings that can be used in evaluating and defending performance decisions. Employees are rated according to specific descriptions of job behavior, which makes it the most legally defensible approach.[8]

The method also is an excellent guide for performance improvement since the evaluation is very specific about what is successful and unsuccessful behavior.

The classic BARS example, which demonstrates this approach, scales the performance factors for Superman. (See Figure 5.7)

BARS requires the development of a range of behavioral statements that show very specific increments of skill. As a result, this tool can be used to orient/train an employee in terms of expected behaviors and then can be used to evaluate performance level very precisely. BARS' most important asset is its ability to present mental pictures of behavior so that an employee can "see" a progression of behavior that moves from incompetent to outstanding. As such, it is an excellent development tool.

Figure 5.7

Guide to Superman performance appraisal

Guide to performance appraisal

Performance degrees

Performance factors (Criteria)	5 Far exceeds job requirements	4 Exceeds job requirements	3 Meets job requirements	2 Needs some improvement	1 Does not meet minimum requirements
Quality	Leaps tall buildings with a single bound	Must take running start to leap tall buildings	Only leaps over short buildings	Crashes into buildings when attempting to jump over	Cannot recognize building at all, much less jump
Timeliness	Faster than a speeding bullet	As fast as a speeding bullet	Not quite as fast as a speeding bullet	Would you believe a slow bullet?	Wounds self with bullet when attempting to shoot gun
Initiative	Stronger than a locomotive	Stronger than a bull elephant	Stronger than a bull	Shoots the bull	Smells like a bull
Adaptability	Walks on water consistently	Walks on water in emergencies	Washes with water	Drinks water	Passes water in emergencies
Communication	Talks with God	Talks with the angels	Talks to self	Argues with self	Loses arguement with self

Figure 5.8

BARS scale

A behaviorally anchored rating scale example for "effective training" is shown below.

Totally unacceptable — incompetent

- Has developed no training procedures.
- Has developed no trained backups.
- Does not determine skill level of trainee.
- Does not assume responsibility for new trainee; delegates to any worker in the unit.

Satisfactory

- Has developed training procedures.
- Has trained backups.
- Provides ongoing training to all employees.
- Assigns experienced employees to coach new employees after determining skill level and providing appropriate training.

Outstanding

- Individualizes training for each employee; plans and schedules training as needed over time.
- Learns and uses contemporary training methods and modes.
- Helps others learn new training techniques and assists them with training.

Another example, a BARS scale for the performance dimension of "effective training," is shown in Figure 5.8.

The drawback to BARS is that it requires a detailed, time-consuming job analysis for each job. Typically a group of employees who perform a job are brought together to identify the range of behaviors (from unacceptable to outstanding) for each critical performance dimension of the job. This is an investment in time and talent that few group practices can afford. Also, BARS may not be flexible enough to include differences between employees with the same job title.

A most useful way to use the BARS technology is to integrate the concept of developing a range of behavioral statements into a criterion-based method, which is one of the three suggested approaches for medical practices.

Suggested approaches

The following approaches can be particularly useful for medical practices. These meet legal requirements for job-relatedness in terms of performance factors and standards, are practical and most important, improve performance. (Samples are provided of each.) The choice depends on practice size, performance philosophy, management traditions and practical considerations (e.g., amount of time available, type of position).

Performance standard method

A performance standard method can be used successfully as both a planning and evaluation tool. It focuses on general job-related factors that are applicable across all employees, or across specific groups.

This type of method is useful in reinforcing the performance factors that are important to a medical practice; e.g., quantity, quality, productivity, patient relations. A definition should be provided for each factor to eliminate misunderstanding about what a factor, such as patient relations, means.

These definitions should be stated in behavioral language. For example, "Patient Relations: Display of respect, patience, helpfulness to patients; friendly manner, appropriate acknowledgment of patient feelings; ability to deal with clients in a nondefensive manner."

As explained in more detail in Chapter Eight, legally it is unacceptable to use personality traits or attitudes as performance criteria. The focus must be on performance factors that are specific and critical to the job.

Once the medical practice has determined the factors it values (e.g., patient relations, productivity), the tool can be used for all employees, both non-exempt and management. This format allows for tailoring to each job. The supervisor should add two to four performance standards and behavioral comments that directly relate to each employee's job. All factors should be discussed and agreed on by the supervisor and the employee.

For example, the supervisor should specify a performance standard for each factor that is defined in terms of the particular job description. Example: For a switchboard operator's position, the performance factor of "Patient Relations" could be coupled with a performance standard that stated: "Answers calls within three rings; greets client with a "smiling," interested tone of voice; connects call correctly on first try within 60 seconds."

Performance measurement standards should be expressed in specific, measurable (quantity, quality, time, cost) terms. In addition, they should be both realistic and challenging. There is nothing more frustrating to an employee than the "impossible dream" and nothing less motivating than an "easy shot."

A simple rating scale can be used with a performance standard tool. A numerical scale is often used (for example, from one to five with one being "unacceptable" and five being "outstanding." A preferred approach is to scale by four categories (for example, does not meet standard, meets standard, above standard, exceeds standard). The word "standard" reinforces the concept of a performance standard of success. It is does not mean average. Rather it means "fully acceptable, competent, proficient"; hitting the mark.

It is useful to note that the use of an odd-numbered scale can cause a tendency to grade in the middle. That is why many performance management experts prefer to use a scale with four points of measurement.

Once the factors and standards have been finalized, the supervisor should use the tool for performance planning. For example, a new employee would not only receive a copy of his or her job description, but also a copy of the performance tool. The supervisor would explain the expectations, and may modify them to fit the new employee's skill/experience level. In the case of a new switchboard operator, this may mean adjusting the standard for the probationary/training period to read: "Connects calls to the right party within 90 seconds" rather than the standard of 60 seconds. This would be the measure of success for the first three months.

With all employees, the tool can be used by the supervisor and employee to plan performance for the next period — to clarify the standard and to agree that it is still appropriate.

The performance standard approach does not take a lot of time to develop or to use, and does not require extensive verbal skills. However, a rating by itself does not inform employees of their deficiencies or motivate them to improve their performance. Therefore, if this method is used, at evaluation time supervisors should be required to include a behavioral, descriptive comment about each factor/standard to clarify the rating. Example: "Employee not only answers calls quickly and connects them correctly, but also takes the initiative to track down staff and/or information for the client."

This approach also requires the assignment of an "importance weight" to each factor. That is, in this tool each factor is assigned a numerical value that reflects its importance in overall job performance. For example, quality might be given a weight of 50 percent. It is important for employees to know how important each factor is or what counts most. Again, this should be discussed at the beginning of each performance period to ensure that the supervisor and employee are in accord on priorities.

This method takes some upfront time to develop in that supervisors must specify significant performance factors, the related standards and the relative weights. However, once the tool is developed, it is very easy to use. It represents a common-sense approach that facilitates effective communication between the supervisor and employee.

Or the group practice could select six to 10 performance standards for each job and then the supervisor adds two to four performance standards that are job specific.

(A sample is provided that can serve as a prototype for medical practices preferring this approach. It presents a list of factors that are generally accepted as significant performance factors and relative weights. See Figures 5.9A and 5.9B)

Figure 5.9A

Sample performance standard evaluation form

Employee ______________________ Date ____________

Title ______________________ Supervisor ____________

Purpose of evaluation: Annual___ 3 Month___ 6 Month___ Other___

Instructions: During the planning session, discuss the performance factors and their definitions. Specify a standard of competence that is relevant to the job description and an importance weight for each factor. Prior to the performance interview provide a comment about each factor. The comment should describe a specific incident(s) in behavioral terms that related directly to the employee's job description. Rate each factor, then multiply by the weight to get the score for the factor. The overall score is a total for all the factors.

Scale	1 Does not meet standard	2 Meets standard	3 Above standard	4 Exceeds standard

JOB KNOWLEDGE: Knowledge of job skills, duties and related work.

Standard: ______________________
Behavioral comment: ______________________
____

Rating_______ Weight: 15 points Score______

QUALITY OF WORK: Organization, effective use of time, accuracy, completeness.

Standard: ______________________
Behavioral comment: ______________________
____

Rating_______ Weight: 15 points Score______

PRODUCTIVITY: Amount of work completed in an average shift.

Standard: ______________________
Behavioral comment: ______________________
____

Rating_______ Weight: 15 points Score______

(Figure 5.9A continued on page 87)

(Figure 5.9A continued from page 86)

Overall rating: ______

Additional supervisor comments: ____________________

Goals for next performance period: ____________________

Employee personal development goals: ____________________

Employee comments: ____________________

Supervisor signature ____________________ Date ________

Employee signature ____________________ Date ________
(Acknowledges employee has reviewed and discussed evaluation)

Figure 5.9B

Sample performance standard evaluation form

Employee ____________________ Date ________

Title ____________________ Supervisor ____________________

Purpose of evaluation: Annual___ 3 Month___ 6 Month___ Other___

Performance Factors

JOB KNOWLEDGE: Skills and abilities necessary to perform job requirements.

Unsatisfactory	Competent	Commendable	Exceptional
❑	❑	❑	❑

Supervisory comments: ____________________

QUALITY OF WORK: Extent to which work performance meets job requirements of accuracy and thoroughness.

Unsatisfactory	Competent	Commendable	Exceptional
❑	❑	❑	❑
Work usually incomplete. Makes obvious and recurring mistakes. Quality usually poor.	Work quality meets acceptable requirements for accuracy and thoroughness.	Exceeds accuracy and thoroughness requirements. Errors infrequent. Needs little supervision.	Outstanding work quality, consistent thoroughness and accuracy. Errors extremely rare.

Supervisory comments: ____________________

(Figure 5.9B continued on page 88)

(Figure 5.9B continued from page 87)

PRODUCTIVITY: Volume of employee output including speed and consistency of work.

Unsatisfactory	Competent	Commendable	Exceptional
❑	❑	❑	❑
Productivity frequently below job requirements. Wastes considerable time. Slow in accomplishing tasks.	Regularly meets productivity requirements. Effective in completing assignments.	Productivity frequently exceeds minimum requirements. Volume of work is high; wastes little time.	Consistently meets or exceeds high productivity expectations. Does more than expected in minimal time.

Supervisory comments: ______________________________

____

Overall rating: ______

Additional supervisor comments:

Goals for next performance period:

Employee personal development goals:

Employee comments:

Supervisor signature ______________________________ Date

Employee signature ______________________________ Date

(Acknowledges employee has reviewed and discussed evaluation)

Criterion-based method

A criterion-based approach is another recommended option. It features more specific descriptions of performance factors. It can be used as both a planning tool at the start/end of the year, and as an evaluation tool.

A criterion approach focuses on clearly defined criteria and standards. That is, a criterion is a specific area of job performance that is used to evaluate an employee's performance, rather than a general performance factor. Example: "Return on investment" is a specific criterion whereas "quality" is a general performance factor.

A performance standard in a criterion-based approach is represented as a series of performance levels. Each level correlates to a particular performance rating for the criterion. Example: A rate of return on investment that is 0 percent to 3 percent might be rated as "does not meet standard"; 4 percent to 5 percent would be "meets standard"; 6 percent to 8 percent would be "above standard"; and 9 percent to 10 percent would be "exceeds standard."

The performance standard in this tool is a yardstick — a performance measurement device that is very specific so that performance expectations are very clear. Again, the measurements should relate to quantity, quality, timeliness, financial parameters and be expressed in numerical or behavioral terms. This will ensure validity and reliability.

When establishing evaluation standards for any performance method, it is important to remember that legally performance standards must reflect two characteristics: reliability and validity.

Reliability is defined as consistency between raters (the standard is so specific that different supervisors using it will evaluate the employee in the same way) and freedom from bias (the standard is objective rather than subjective).

Validity is defined as having criteria that are job related (for example, typing speed and accuracy for a clerical position) and standards that actually reflect differences in performance (for example, the standard for typing speed ranges from "does not meet standard" — 35 to 40 wpm — to "meets standard — 50 to 60 wpm — to "above standard" — 65 to 70 wpm — to "exceeds standard" — 75 to 85 wpm).

Some criteria may not be appropriately quantifiable such as verbal communication. The quantity of words spoken could be measured, or the amount of time used. However, a more meaningful measure would be the quality of verbal communication as defined in behavioral terms, such as, this "exceeds standard" description; "Can speak extemporaneously to a group with little notice on a variety of topics." In this case, behavioral statements can serve as the performance standard and the BARS technique can be used to develop them.

There are five steps involved in developing criteria and standards for performance evaluation are (See Figure 5.10):[9]

Figure 5.10

Performance criteria/ standards steps

The steps involved in developing criteria and standards for performance evaluation are:

STEP ONE: Criteria generation

STEP TWO: Criteria selection

STEP THREE: Criteria definition

STEP FOUR: Standards generation

STEP FIVE: Standards rating

Step 1 — Criteria generation/brainstorming/ listing: Job incumbents and supervisors identify criteria related to the incumbents' job that might be included in a performance evaluation.

Step 2 — Criteria selection: The results from step one are combined into a single list and returned to the incumbents and supervisors who then select between 10 and 25 criteria that they feel are the most important to their job and that should be included in a performance evaluation.

Step 3 — Criteria definition: Small groups are formed, each of which is responsible for defining a few of the criteria selected in step two. Once all groups have defined their criteria, definitions are exchanged to permit review and possible revision by those affected by the evaluation.

Step 4 — Standards generation/brainstorming/listing: Job incumbents and supervisors are asked to give examples of behaviors related to levels of performance within each criterion.

Step 5 — Standards rating: The results for each criterion from step four are combined into a single list in random order. Incumbents and supervisors rate each behavioral example on a scale of one to four as follows:

1 — does not meet standard
2 — meets standard
3 — above standard
4 — exceeds standard

This approach takes considerable time and effort to develop. However, it is a most useful exercise for the job incumbents and supervisors in terms of identifying successful behavior via very clear criteria and standards. It also serves as an excellent training tool to establish clear expectations for new employees. (A sample format for building a criterion-based performance evaluation tool is provided. See Figure 5.11 on the following page.)

Goal-setting method

A goal-setting system can be used that involves negotiations between the supervisor and employee to establish performance objectives. It is used at the beginning of a performance period, which might be the probationary/ training period or a complete year. One well-known

Figure 5.11

Sample criterion-based performance evaluation form

Employee ______________________________ Date ______________

Title ______________________________ Supervisor ______________

Purpose of evaluation: Annual___ 3 Month___ 6 Month___ Other___

Instructions: The form specifies one criterion that is applicable to all employees and the related performance standard. In the planning session, the supervisor and employee should list and define other criteria that are specifically related to the employee's job and develop standards that reflect four levels of performance for each criterion (does not meet standard, meets standard, above standard, exceeds standard). Prior to the performance review, a rating should be given to each factor and a behavioral comment provided. The comment should describe a specific incident(s) that reflects the level of performance.

Scale	1 Does not meet standard	2 Meets standard	3 Above standard	4 Exceeds standard

CRITERION: Patient relations: Display of respect, patience, helpfulness to patients, friendly manner, appropriate acknowledgement of patients' feelings.

Did Not Meet	Meets	Above	Exceeds
Clients complain about employee.	Clients generally compliment employee.	Clients often compliment employee.	Clients rate employee highly.
Employee has difficulty dealing with clients.	Employee maintains rapport.	Employee has satisfied clients.	Employee takes initiative to help client.

Rating:_________

CRITERION: ______________________________

Standard: ______________________________

Rating: ______________________________

Comment: ______________________________

(List as many criteria as appropriate.)

OVERALL PERFORMANCE

Rate the employee's overall job performance during the evaluation period:

Does not meet standard____ Meets standard____ Above standard____ Exceeds standard____

Comments: ______________________________

____

List other significant accomplishments attained during the evaluation period.

____

____

____

____

____

(Figure 5.11 continued on page 92)

(Figure 5.11 continued from page 91)

GOALS: List specific performance and development goals for the next evaluation period.

____

____

____

EMPLOYEE COMMENTS: ____

____

____

____

____

Supervisor signature ______________________________ Date __________

Employee signature ______________________________ Date __________
(Acknowledges employee has reviewed and discussed evaluation)

technique is management by objectives (MBO). It involves mutual goal-setting between supervisors and employees. These goals specify the results an employee should aim to accomplish within a predetermined time period.[6]

The MBO approach usually involves:

- job review and agreement by supervisor and employee;
- development of performance standards by both;
- reality check to ensure that attainment of the objectives are achievable (resources are available, the employee has control over the outcome); and
- ongoing discussions concerning the employee's performance in regard to the pre-established objectives.

MBO focuses on the organization's goals and objectives, and this is its main strength. It is directly tied to the strategic plan/annual plan so the employee is very aware of how his or her performance will make a difference to the organization's success. In addition, employee input is stressed to improve commitment and performance.

A major drawback in the MBO process is that it may be useful for management positions, but may not work well for other types of jobs. Example: It may be difficult to tie the performance of a medical records clerk to specific organizational objectives.

In addition, the MBO approach may concentrate too heavily on results, ignoring the methods required to

> “We use a two-page form with space for narrative about developmental goals and training needs. We recommend that supervisors provide the form to employees so they can evaluate themselves before the performance review. They often are harder on themselves than their supervisors.”
>
> *(MGMA member, medium-sized clinic)*

achieve the objectives. That is, it may become a matter of “winning the war, but killing all the troops in the process.” It also is a time-consuming process since the supervisor must invest considerable time negotiating with each employee.

Variations of MBO that use goal-setting, but are less directly tied to specific organizational objectives, offer considerable merit to medical practices. A goal-setting format that works well is one focused on Major Accountabilities (or Key Responsibilities or Key Result Areas) related to the job description. In this approach, three to six major accountabilities are identified and then the supervisor and employee negotiate expected results in terms of objectives and measurable standards. These also may be weighted to indicate priority.

Example: The job description of an ultrasound technologist may include the maintenance of ultrasound equipment as a major accountability. Expected results would be negotiated in terms of goals and measurable standards, as shown below:

> **Goal:** To ensure that ultrasound equipment is in working order.
>
> **Standards:** Inspects equipment on a daily basis; schedules manufacturer’s inspection quarterly; ensures backup equipment is available within two hours.

In addition to specific results-oriented goals, this type of approach can include a section on job-related behaviors. For example, teamwork, patient relations, flexibility, following through on commitments, responsiveness, problem-solving, communication or other factors affecting the manner in which work is performed.

Adding on this type of behavioral focus sends a clear message that the method of achieving the result — how it is done, is equally as important as what is done. This eliminates one of the failures associated with MBO, which focuses only on results.

An accountability type of approach is simple, straightforward and takes little time since it is directly tied to the job description. It also takes advantage of the opportunity to gain the employee’s commitment and to improve performance through the goal-setting discussion.

> “We do performance evaluations three times a year. We use a one-page form that the employee fills out. The items vary each time; e.g., positive problem-solving, use of time, patient relations. The scale is "always do it, most of the time do it, sometimes do it, plan to improve." Then the employee meets with the supervisor for a formal discussion.”
>
> *(MGMA member, small, rural clinic)*

The method is particularly appropriate for use with new employees since it spotlights the job responsibilities and allows for setting accountabilities, goals and standards to reasonable, realistic levels for the initial performance period. Then goals and standards can be increased as the employee reaches certain milestones. It is useful with every level of employee, and is particularly appropriate at the management level where the focus on results and accountabilities is of major importance. (A sample of the goal-setting approach on page 95. See Figure 5.12.)

Non-exempt vs. manager/ supervisor forms

Some medical practices use the same tool for all employees regardless of job function or exempt/non-exempt status; that is, exempt or not exempt from the overtime requirements specified in the Fair Labor Standards Act. Others will identify key performance factors that are mandatory for every employee, for example, patient relations, and then add on other performance factors for specific jobs or levels. Using separate forms for management and nonmanagement staff is recommended. This is an effective way of reinforcing performance factors that are management in nature.

Or a fill-in-the blank approach can be used that calls for:

- major accountabilities, which are tailored to each employee's job description;
- job-related behaviors that are critical for all employees; and
- management-related factors that are just applicable for supervisors/managers. (The format provided in Figure 5.13 on page 97 includes a supervisor's section.)

Each group practice must decide on the management factors most important to them. However, classic factors include leadership, creativity/innovation, decision making, fiscal responsibility, strategic planning. Again, it is critical to define each factor.

Figure 5.12

Sample goal-setting performance evaluation form

Employee ______________________ Date __________

Title ______________________ Supervisor __________

Purpose of evaluation: Annual___ 3 Month___ 6 Month___ Other___

Instructions: This form should be used to (a) develop a performance plan for the employee and (b) to track/evaluate performance. Responsibilities, goals and priorities are to be mutually agreed upon by the supervisor and employee in the planning session. Accomplishments should be noted prior to the performance review by the employee and then discussed with the supervisor.

I. JOB RESPONSIBILITIES: List major job responsibilities in priority order.

II. PERFORMANCE GOALS: Indicate specific, desired results to be accomplished. Goals should specify required quality, quantity, timeliness, cost or any other appropriate measures. Completion dates should be included.

III. ACCOMPLISHMENTS: Show specific evidence of achievement related to each goal. This section is filled out by the employee prior to review with supervisor.

IV. SUPERVISOR'S EVALUATION: Indicates the supervisor's assessment of performance related to each goal and a rating given for each goal.

1	2	3	4
Does not meet goal	**Meets goal**	**Above goal**	**Exceeds goal**

V. GENERAL PERFORMANCE FACTORS: Indicates assessment of supervisor related to employee's performance behaviors using the same scale as above. The supervisor also must support the rating with a comment about a specific observation(s) of the behavior.

Initiative: Sees beyond the immediate assignment and acts on opportunities and problem areas.

Rating:_____Observation: ______________________

Follow through: Sees that objectives and related action steps are followed through to completion.

Rating:_____Observation: ______________________

Interpersonal relations: Communicates, listens, presents self and one's ideas effectively.

Rating:_____Observation: ______________________

(Figure 5.12 continued on page 96)

(Figure 5.12 continued from page 95)

Teamwork: Works effectively with others to maximize attainment of group goals.

Rating:_____Observation: ______________________________

Patient relations: Displays respect, patience, helpfulness to patients, friendly manner, appropriate acknowledge of patient's feelings.

Rating:_____Observation: ______________________________

VI: SUPERVISOR COMPETENCIES: Applies to supervisory employees only.

Planning: Identifies desired outcomes and develops long- and short-range steps for accomplishing them.

Rating:_____Observation: ______________________________

Controlling: Establishes standards and monitors people or processes to maintain such standards.

Rating:_____Observation: ______________________________

Team building: Takes a leadership role in developing a cohesive, effective work group.

Rating:_____Observation: ______________________________

Developing employees: Trains employees, gives instructions and feedback, coaches and counsels, appraises employees frequently, delegates responsibility.

Rating:_____Observation: ______________________________

VII. OVERALL PERFORMANCE SUMMARY:

Rating:_____Comments: ______________________________

____

____

VIII. DEVELOPMENT PLANNING

Employee strengths: ______________________________

Improvement areas: ______________________________

Development plan: ______________________________

Supervisor signature: ______________________________ Date______________

Employee signature: ______________________________ Date______________

(Acknowledges employee has reviewed and discussed evaluation)

Figure 5.13

Sample mid-year performance evaluation form

Employee ______________________________ Date ______________

Title ______________________ Supervisor ____________________

Instructions: Complete this form six months after the performance plan has been developed to check on progress. Answer the questions and make modifications to the performance plan, if appropriate.

1. Have the employee's major job responsibilities changed since the expectations were established?
2. Should goals be changed, revised or expanded?
3. Outline appropriate changes and attach to performance plan, or complete a new performance plan.
4. Indicate year-to-date performance results for each responsibility, goal or accountability.
5. Describe plans for improvement, if needed.
6. Supervisor comments:
7. Employee comments:

Supervisor signature ______________________________ Date

Employee signature ______________________________ Date
(Acknowledges employee has reviewed and discussed evaluation)

Other options

With any performance management process, it is worthwhile to include quarterly or mid-year reviews. These are especially helpful when the goal-setting approach is used. In this case, the form should include an extra sheet that would cover such factors to consider as:

- job responsibility changes;
- goal changes;
- performance plan changes;
- year-to-date performance results;
- improvement plans;

> “Our evaluation is based on self-evaluation and feedback from co-workers; e.g., 'Are the programmer services provided by Joe satisfactory?' We also contact physicians in writing; e.g., 'I'd like your input on Joe's evaluation. How do you rate his responsiveness, quality of work, effectiveness, dependability, accuracy?' They can respond with comments or give a ranking of 1 to 5. Physicians don't like to spend time doing this and/or they are uncomfortable doing evaluations. The benefit of the approach is that the staffers know upfront that others will be assessing their performance. This gives a competitive edge to the process.”
>
> *(MGMA member, large clinic)*

- supervisor comments;
- employee comments;
- employee and supervisor signatures; and
- date.

Performance reviews during the year provide performance "insurance" in several ways. First, they help the supervisor and employee check to see if the world changed since the plan was developed. Often, a plan put in place at the start of a year is totally obsolete by mid-year because job responsibilities have changed — but goals and expectations have not. The plan becomes irrelevant and as result, erodes the very meaning of performance planning and evaluation.

Second, the sessions allow the employee and supervisor to look closely at results to date and to make corrections or improvements before it is too late. There is nothing sadder or sillier than to wait to the end of the year to check on progress. Medical practice managers certainly refuse to do that when tracking financial performance. They demand financial statements every month to ensure they are on target with budgetary expectations.

In certain cases, quarterly reviews are especially recommended. This is a traditional approach with new employees (that is, the introductory period review). However, it can also be used very successfully when an employee is working on a new project, or trying to develop a new skill. And more frequent reviews are imperative when supervisors are working with employees who have performance problems, as discussed in a later chapter.

Another option that is worthwhile is self-assessment. There are two standard techniques used with this approach. One is to have employees evaluate themselves on the performance evaluation form prior to the performance review. They then compare their evaluations with those of the supervisor, who also has filled out a form. This approach stimulates a very meaningful discussion, especially if there are significant discrepancies between the supervisor's and employee's evaluations. The final ratings/comments are put on a third copy of the form after the discussion.

A second approach is to give the employee a generic self-assessment form that asks questions about (See Figure 5.14):

- major contributions;
- career goals;
- long-range goals;
- skill/knowledge training;

Figure 5.14

Sample self-appraisal worksheet

These questions will help you prepare for your performance evaluation discussion with your supervisor. Think about your performance, your progress and your plans for future development.

1. What abilities does my job require?
2. What do I like best about my job? The least?
3. What were my specific accomplishments since the last evaluation period?
4. Which goals or standards did I fall short of meeting? Why?
5. How could my supervisor help me to do a better job?
6. Is there anything the organization or my supervisor does that hinders my effectiveness?
7. What job changes would improve my effectiveness?
8. Does my current job utilize all my capabilities? How could I become more productive for the organization?
9. What personal career/development goals do I have?
10. Do I need more experience or training in any aspect of my current job? How could it be accomplished?
11. What have I done since my last evaluation to prepare myself for more responsibility?
12. What new goals and standards should be established for the next evaluation period? Which old ones should be modified or deleted?

Other comments: ______________________________

____

____

____

Employee ______________________________ Date ______________

Title ______________________________

Supervisor ______________________________

> "Now that we are beginning to move into TQM, we are moving to modify the performance system. We expect to take away the grades and to have more room for narrative about each category. We will focus on teamwork and customer satisfaction, things that were not necessarily priorities in the past."
>
> *(MGMA member, medium-sized clinic)*

- required assistance;
- major strengths;
- improvement areas; and
- other comments.

Whatever self-evaluation method is used, its purpose is to inspire the employee to think ahead about the interview, to evaluate his or her own performance, to prepare for a significant discussion. This gives the employee not only a sense of control over the discussion, but also a sense of responsibility for it — this is a participatory approach rather than a parent-child approach.

Design review

Once a medical practice has decided on the type of approach that best fits its situation and has developed a prototype, it should be reviewed. As noted before, if a Performance Focus task force has been organized, it will provide an appropriate mix of employees, supervisors and managers who can review the draft.

If such a task force is not in place, the prototype should still be reviewed by a variety of individuals. Senior management, of course, should review it carefully because of its critical implications to morale and productivity. The board of directors should participate in the review and approval process. The organization's legal counsel should also review it to ensure it is defensible.

In addition, supervisors of the medical practice should have an opportunity to have input. And ideally, a sampling of employees should be invited to serve as reviewers.

Revisions, pre-test, finalizing

After the review, the suggested changes should be carefully analyzed. If they are warranted, the next step is to modify the system accordingly.

The final "insurance" step is to run a pilot test of the process. One way to do this is to ask three supervisors of different departments to use the system for a specified period; i.e., three months. Then their input on its real-life application should be reviewed and incorporated into the process. The focus on this point is moving from the theoretical to such key questions as:

- Is it understandable?
- Is it time efficient?
- Is it successful (Does it do what it is supposed to do — define and improve performance)?

Once the "bugs" are out of the system, it should be finalized. This step typically involves not only printing the forms, but also developing a manual for supervisors that "walks them through the process" step by step. In addition, much briefer information about the process should be developed for the employees' handbook. These steps are the beginning of the implementation stage, as described in the next chapter.

Summing up

In conclusion, there is no one perfect tool or one right way for a medical practice to develop a performance management process. Each must determine what best fits their situation.

When making a choice, the most important consideration is to ensure that the approach is job related and behaviorally based.

NOTE: The sample forms presented in this chapter are intended to serve only as guides when medical practices are designing their own forms. Therefore, they are presented in an abbreviated fashion.

FOOTNOTES

[1]*Courtney Price, Alys Novak.* Health Care Innovation and Venture Trends. *Albany, N.Y.: Delmar Publishers, 1992, p. 40.*

[2]*Courtney Price.* The Group Practice Personnel Policies Manual. *Denver, Colo.: Medical Group Management Association, 1991, p. V-17.*

[3]*H. John Bernardin, Richard W. Beatty.* Performance Appraisal: Assessing Human Resources at Work. *Belmont, Calif.: Wadsworth, Inc., 1984, p. 191.*

[4]*Courtney Price, Bruce Stickler.* Personnel Postscript. *Medical Group Management Association, Spring 1990, p. 5.*

[5]*ibid, p. 5.*

[6]*ibid, p. 7.*

[7]*ibid, p. 6.*

[8]*ibid, p. 4.*

[9]*Courtney Price.* Summary of the Development of Criteria and Standards for Performance Evaluation. *Seminar presentation, 1986.*

Implementing the process

Chapter Six

The management team of a medium-sized medical practice was feeling very proud of itself. After observing the trend toward revising performance management systems, it had hired a consultant to develop a new process for the organization. The consultant turned in a final product that seemed right on the mark. The CEO scheduled an all-staff meeting and proudly announced the new process. Each supervisor was given a set of forms and told to "go to it." In varying degrees they did, with results that varied from not so bad, to very bad. Supervisors "forgot" to do the upfront planning; they didn't follow the procedures; they neglected to turn in their paperwork. And the employees grumbled about "another fad." Result: morale decreased, performance remained unchanged.

Once the system has been pre-tested and revised accordingly, it is time to implement the system thoughtfully or all the good work that was put into development goes down the drain. A checklist of the steps to follow includes (See Figure 6.1 on the following page):

Figure 6.1

Process implementation steps

Once the performance management process has been designed and approved, it needs to be implemented following these steps:

✔system procedures;

✔user orientation;

✔supervisory training;

✔performance period designation;

✔interview schedule;

✔initial performance evaluations;

✔development planning;

✔performance discussions;

✔feedback schedules;

✔system review;

✔results monitoring; and

✔revision.

- prepare and disseminate systems procedures;
- develop and deliver user orientation;
- develop and deliver supervisory training;
- establish performance/evaluation period;
- schedule interviews;
- discuss performance evaluation;
- discuss development plans;
- make personnel decisions;
- schedule time for feedback;
- review system;
- monitor results; and
- revise (if necessary).

System procedures

To ensure effective implementation of the performance management process (PMP), it is important to document it in terms of policies and procedures. These documents should become part of the organization's policy/procedure manual. Some medical practices may have one manual that includes all policies (general guiding principles) established by the board and senior management, as well as the accompanying procedures (the detailed steps for carrying out the policies).

Other medical practices may place all its human resource/personnel documents in a separate handbook. In addition, these policies and procedures may be included in a "Supervisor's Manual" as well as summarized in an "Employee Handbook."

An "Employee Handbook" classically contains general information about the organization and specific information about personnel policies, such as salary/wage schedule, benefits options, dress code, hours of business, smoking restrictions ... and general information about the performance management process.

Usually this manual is given to every employee at the time of hire and updated regularly, usually annually. However, if the performance management process is introduced during the year, all of these materials will need to be revised accordingly.

As discussed before, a vital component of the process is the philosophy statement, which states the medical practice's beliefs about performance management. This should be followed by the organization's policy statement, which has been approved by the board. Both of these statements should be included in all the manuals.

Once these bottom-line statements have been developed, the designers of the performance management process can develop the related procedures. Typically, procedures are developed related to:

- process cycle (timing of planning, evaluation, feedback, salary decisions, report to management);
- responsibilities (management, supervisor, employee);
- salary decisions (relationship with evaluations, timing link);
- training (general orientation, supervisory training);
- documentation (reporting/filing of results);
- employee materials (copies of plan and evaluation kept by employee);
- job changes (personnel movement during the year);
- terminations (employee resignation, discharge); and
- grievance (appeal procedure).

To get started, it would be useful to review the examples of performance evaluation policies and procedures.[1]

Here's one example:

"The policy of the ABC Clinic is to plan, review and evaluate each employee's performance periodically in an objective, consistent and uniform manner. The plan and evaluation consists of a written performance plan according to a standard format, with discussion of the plan and evaluation with the employee.

The following procedures should be used to implement this policy:

- At the beginning of the performance period, the supervisor and employee should establish performance objectives and standards and document them.

- During the performance period, the supervisor should provide constant feedback on performance. The employee also should be responsible for monitoring and correcting performance.

- The performance evaluations are conducted by the employee's immediate supervisor with input from the employee.

- The performance evaluation is based on the job description, productivity goals, experience and training of the employee.

- Information derived from performance evaluations is used to determine the employee's eligibility for merit salary increases, promotion, transfer, layoff and retention, and to identify training needs of the employee.

- Performance evaluation is conducted at least annually and copies of this report are submitted to the human resources department.

- Performance evaluations are completed:

    - after the first six months of employment;

    - on each anniversary date of employment thereafter;

    - when the employee is transferred or promoted to a new job;

    - upon the employee's termination; and

  - whenever the overall evaluation is below standard; then, additional evaluations are required every three months (or if necessary, more frequently) until the employee receives a satisfactory rating.

- The employee's performance planning and evaluation are a permanent part of the employee's record.

- Supervisors are encouraged to keep informal records of significant events concerning the employee's job performance.

- Performance planning and evaluation should be used to encourage better communication between the employee and supervisor.

- Following completion by the supervisor, each performance evaluation is reviewed by the appropriate department director to assure objectivity and fairness before discussing the evaluation with the employee. After the evaluation has been approved by the department director, the supervisor discusses the evaluation with the employee.

- At the time of the performance evaluation interview, the employee is given the opportunity to discuss concerns, correct inaccuracies and make written comments concerning any aspect of the evaluation. The written evaluation then is forwarded to the human resources department to include in the employee's personnel file.

- Each supervisor uses these guidelines to prepare and conduct the performance evaluation:

  - Evaluate each employee's performance on the basis of job-related criteria and productivity goals;

  - Evaluate each employee on the basis of overall performance since the previous evaluation, and do not give in to recent events;

  - Maintain a balance between praise and criticism, acting as a counselor, not a judge;

  - Plan each performance evaluation interview to make it as positive and constructive as possible.

The interview should be private and confidential. Schedule it far enough in advance to allow for pertinent discussions and revisions when necessary. Tell the employee in advance of the scheduled interview;

- Use the performance evaluation to plan goals for the next period and encourage improvement when necessary;
- Note deficiencies and suggest steps for improvements;
- Allow the employee to talk freely about the job, encourage his/her input and listen;
- Check the employee's progress, commend improvement and take appropriate action when improvement has not been made;
- If the performance evaluation contains a rating which the employee feels is unfair or unjustified and the matter has not been resolved to the employee's satisfaction during the interview, the employee may file a grievance; and
- Supervisors are encouraged to regularly discuss an employee's job performance on an informal basis." (*Source: The Group Practice Personnel Policies Manual*)

Policies and procedures similar to these that are developed by each medical practice form the basis for both user orientation and supervisory training. (See Figure 6.2 on the following page.)

User orientation

In this case "user" is defined as anyone who will be impacted by the PMP. This covers every level in the medical practice, including senior management, supervisors and employees.

Most, if not all, of the management team will have been involved in the design phase of the process. Initially, they

Figure 6.2

Sample trial period policies

Each medical practice should develop policies related to the "probation/trial period" for new employees, as this example illustrates.

To acclimate new employees to ABC Clinic and to the employee's position, your first six months of employment are considered a trial period. If you successfully complete this period, you will become a regular employee, eligible for the various benefits set forth in this handbook. Like regular employees, trial employees are employees at will and may be terminated at any time without cause and without prior notice.

In case of promotions, demotions or transfers within the organization, an employee who, in the sole judgment of management, is not successful in his or her new position can be removed from that job at any time during the probationary period. The employee will be allowed to return to his or her former job, if it is available or to any other comparable available job for which the employee is qualified.

will have provided guidance and objectives as well as participated in the development of the philosophy and policy statement. Some will have been assigned to work with the Performance Focus task force/designers; others will have been given the opportunity to review the prototype.

Once the PMP is finalized and ready for launch, the orientation for these individuals, at a managers' meeting, should focus on the broad perspective of "what this will mean" to other users. That is, the emphasis must be on the supervisors who will be the key players in making it a successful process and the employees who also must be major participants if the PMP is to result in productivity and performance improvements.

Not only will the management team need to understand how the PMP will operate, they must also be prepared to "walk the talk," or serve as promoters of the process through daily demonstrations of "how we do it here." They should model the process with their subordinates — the supervisors — and coach the supervisors in using the PMP effectively with their subordinates. Most of all, they should monitor the supervisors' use of the process.

Supervisors, as noted several times, are the key users. Thus, their orientation should occur in two parts:

- They should be oriented generally about the PMP in a supervisors' meeting.

- During this meeting, they should be alerted about the in-depth orientation they will receive in the supervisory training.

- There should be a step-by-step introduction to the process, with opportunities to practice key components.

Initial orientation of employees to the PMP can occur in several ways, and a combination is recommended. If possible, an all-employee meeting will be held to launch the process. Management will introduce the PMP briefly and provide written information about it. This is an appropriate time to pass out the newly revised "Employee Handbook" with the updated section on performance management.

Ideally, employees would already be aware that a new process was in the works through previous announcements about the Performance Focus task force/design effort. And some of them would have been part of this team. Additionally, during the design period, hopefully employees would have been surveyed to learn their opinions about the present process.

The meeting then becomes an opportunity to thank employees for their input and to affirm that "we heard your preferences and here is your process." There would be a short period for questions and answers led by the human resource professional and or administrator, who will be named as the managers of the system. They will also serve as the main information resource about the PMP.

In addition, employees would be encouraged to save their detailed questions for a meeting with their supervisors. Each supervisor would meet with his or her work unit to go through the PMP again and to discuss how and when it will be implemented for this group. Supervisors should reinforce the idea of a performance partnership. "This is our process ... we'll do it together. I'm your resource, your coach."

By using this combination, employees will be given a three-fold introduction to the process:

- management overview;
- written reference; and
- supervisor's details.

> “What's unique in group practices is the determination of who's involved in performance management; e.g., direct supervisor, physicians. The employee must be responsive to both the supervisor and to the group physicians. So we must expand our idea of the team that evaluates an employee. This requires a great deal of training and is difficult to do.”
>
> *(MGMA member, medium-sized clinic)*

To supplement this approach, articles about the process could be published in the employee newsletter if one is available. The point should be made that the process is new and may need to be modified after a period of use. Again, employee input should be sought and directed to the human resource specialist and/or administrator.

Employees who join the medical practice after the launch, should be introduced to the PMP in their regular orientation by the human resource specialist. Then supervisors should use the "Employee Handbook" as a reference when developing the initial performance plan with new employees so they understand how the process is applied.

For smaller groups, the introduction of the PMP can be handled simply in a regular staff meeting with current employees, and then one-on-one with each new employee.

Supervisory training

For larger group practices, an excellent method for training supervisors about the performance management process is to develop and use a "Supervisor's Manual" that describes the PMP and walks the supervisor through it. It can then serve as not only the training tool, but also as the daily reference.

Such a manual would typically include the following sections (sample information is also shown).

Letter from the CEO

This section classically serves to reinforce the commitment of the chief executive officer of the medical practice to the process, such as:

> *"We have developed this manual to describe our performance management process (PMP). As the process was being designed, we received several ideas*

from our employees and many were built into the final product. We believe that these performance guidelines will significantly improve our understanding of how to deliver truly excellent service for all our customers.

"We have aimed to provide you with as comprehensive a manual as possible so that you will have the information you need to be as effective as possible. The supervisor, as the person who has daily contact with the employee, has the best opportunity to observe, guide and coach performance. Thus, we hope you will become thoroughly familiar with the system. A good working knowledge of performance management will make you more effective in encouraging high performance from your employees and this, in turn, will improve your performance.

"In order to successfully serve our customers, we must manage our workforce effectively. We need to give employees the clarity of purpose that will enable them to succeed. In this manual, you'll find many ideas that will help you be more effective as a manager. Be willing to use them. Willingness to develop your supervisory skills through training should make this a better workplace."

Background of the process

This section includes a discussion of how and why the performance management process was developed and typically spotlights the goal of the program and its objectives, such as:

Goal

To carefully plan and carefully evaluate employee job behavior in order to improve performance.

Objectives

- Everyone who uses or is affected by the process will know how the process works;

- Evaluations are based solely on how well employees perform their jobs. Through job descriptions, the evaluations are tied as closely as possible to specific features of jobs;

- Both supervisors and employees participate in goal setting, feedback and evaluation processes;
- The process takes into account changes in job duties and responsibilities;
- The process not only improves performance, but also contributes to personal and professional development;
- The process provides a solid basis for arriving at effective and supportable personnel decisions such as recruiting, promoting, training, transferring, compensating and so forth; and
- The process does not involve too much paperwork or time.

General description

This section outlines the key features of the performance management process, explaining its design, how it is intended to work, and the supervisor's role in the process.

The process:

- is more than a rating form.
- allows tailoring to jobs being evaluated.
- evaluates employees in several ways.
- begins with performance planning.
- continues throughout the year.
- has a cycle.
- helps supervisors explain and defend their evaluations.
- follows the employee throughout their careers with the organization.

Performance planning

This section discusses how performance planning is done, based on the format chosen; (performance standard method, criterion-based form, goal-setting approach). If performance factors such as quality are emphasized in the format, the planning session includes a full discussion of not only what quality is, but how to achieve it.

If performance objectives are also covered in the format, the discussion is more focused on specific success targets; for example, increasing productivity or decreasing client complaints by a certain percent.

Performance factors and objectives are elaborated on in this section so supervisors understand:

> “We have a training program once a year about our performance management system which is given by the human resource staff. We emphasize what we would like to see accomplished, the steps of performance management, such as planning goals, communicating goals, how to apply the system, how to respond to progress/lack of, how to monitor performance, how to correct performance. In these sessions and others, we are always discussing new ways to do performance management.”
>
> *(MGMA member, medium-sized clinic)*

- what they are;
- how they are used;
- when to schedule the planning;
- how to plan with employees;
- how to utilize job descriptions and organizational goals;
- how to include weights, priorities, time percentages (where appropriate);
- how to establish accountabilities/key responsibility areas (where appropriate);
- how to plan for feedback; and
- how to document the plan.

Tracking performance during the year

This section of the manual provides suggestions for monitoring employee performance and giving appropriate feedback throughout the year.

Topics covered include:

- why progress should be tracked;
- how performance objectives can change;
- how employees should participate in ongoing reviews;
- how performance should be documented; and

- how feedback should be given.

The performance planning step is the most important part of the performance management process since it clarifies expectations and sets success targets. The value of this step will be eroded without the second step of ongoing feedback. Employees need to consistently know if they are on or off target. Waiting until the performance year-end interview for feedback significantly reduces the possibility of top performance.

Performance evaluation

This section of the manual describes the steps to be followed in completing the employee's evaluation. It typically includes information on:

- who completes the form;
- what biases should be avoided;
- what procedures should be followed;
- what type of documentation should be used;
- how employee self-evaluation information can be utilized; and
- how performance information should be summarized.

This section focuses on helping supervisors see the completion of the form as an important summing-up step in the process, but not as the only or the most important step of the process. If prior steps of planning and tracking — have been done well, the completion of the form is basically a ritual, a fitting conclusion for a successful journey toward successful performance management by both "partners."

The interview session

This section of the manual provides suggestions to use in conducting the evaluation conference. This conference is the most challenging part of the evaluation process since it requires careful preparation by the supervisor to ensure each employee is treated fairly and with consideration. With proper planning, the result should be positive for both.

Usually this section includes information on:

- what is the evaluation conference?
- why have an evaluation conference?
- who participates in the conference?
- how should supervisors prepare? and
- what can supervisors do to make the conference more successful?

Sample forms

The manual also includes copies of the recommended forms to use in the process, including full instructions on how and when to use them.

Appendix

Frequently a "Supervisor's Manual" will also include detailed information on:

- performance evaluation and the law;
- management tips;
- common pitfalls in performance planning and evaluation;
- behavioral modification tips;
- job analysis guide;
- job description guide; and
- performance interview guide.

The supervisory training using this manual as the "text" is generally conducted by the PMP designers and/or the human resource professional. It is useful to have the session kicked off by the chief executive officer, as a strong endorsement of the system.

This training not only should be scheduled when the PMP is introduced, but also should become a regular component of the overall training curriculum for new supervisors. In addition, each year supervisors should have a review/update on the process before the planning period.

Managers should document this training to ensure it takes place. They should also discuss the training with their supervisors to ensure they understand how to use the system.

Evaluation period

The performance management process should have a defined cycle that is clear to everyone in terms of a beginning and an end. In establishing such a cycle, these questions should be asked:

- Should the cycle coincide with the calendar year, fiscal year, annual planning period?
- Should the cycle be the same for all employees or be linked to the employee's anniversary date?
- Should the cycle be linked to the salary cycle?
- Should there be a new employee cycle?
- Should there be a performance problem cycle?

If a medical practice chooses to use a goal-setting format, linking the performance cycle with the calendar/fiscal/annual planning period should occur. In this case, performance objectives can be established that give each employee "a piece of the action." His or her contribution to overall objectives is clear and is very motivational, particularly if the medical practice has a profit sharing or other incentive system. At the end of the year, the employee's evaluation can be linked very specifically both to individual results and organizational results.

If there is no specific link between the organizational goals and the employee's goals, it is not necessary for the performance cycle to be the same for all employees. In this case, staggering the planning/evaluations is acceptable and can allow more individual attention. Frequently, this type of staggering is done based on employee anniversary date, which is established once the probationary or training period is successfully concluded.

As will be discussed in more detail in Chapter Ten, most performance management specialists strongly recommend not linking performance reviews with salary reviews. The basic reason: If employees are thinking about money in the performance interview, they are not hearing comments about performance.

If the medical practice does link the two reviews, the cycle must be in sync with the budgetary cycle or when raises are scheduled to impact the financial condition of the organization.

Another option is to schedule the performance interview to discuss performance and then shortly after, schedule another meeting to discuss salary changes.

When considering performance planning and evaluation for the new employee, it is important to adjust the performance cycle. First, it is critical to get the employee off to the right start by setting performance expectations as part of the initial orientation and training. Thus, a performance plan must be established for an "introductory" period.

Historically, employers have established a probationary or training period for new hires and/or employees who have been promoted. This period provides an opportunity for new employees to evaluate their new work situations and for management to evaluate job performance and suitability for employment. More specifically, this period should be used to assess the knowledge, skills and abilities of new employees to determine if they can successfully perform specific job duties.[2]

There is a trend today to substitute different terms for the word "probation," which has a negative, punitive connotation. Instead, consider using words like trial, introductory, provisional, training or orientation period. Again, the intent should be to focus on effective performance and on giving the new employee special attention during this period as a means of ensuring success.

For the new employee, an introductory period allows him or her to learn the job, ask questions about job duties and responsibilities, ensure he or she fits the position and the employer, and get to know the people with whom he or she will be working. Of course, the employee always has the option, at this time or any time, to leave if there does not seem to be a fit.

Another use of an introductory period by health care employers is whenever an employee transfers or is promoted. Again, the employer should have a policy about what happens if the employee does not fit the new position. Will he or she be able to return to the former job or to bid on vacant positions? This policy should be stated clearly in the personnel policies manual.

An introductory period should be long enough to allow the employer to assess the employee's ability and to conduct periodic evaluations. Most medical practices establish either a three- or six-month introductory period for non-exempt employees.

Six to 12 months is a more appropriate length for evaluating new professional and management employees. There should also be the option to extend the introductory period if the employee is making progress but has not yet reached a satisfactory performance level.

During the introductory period, in most states, the employee may be terminated at any time, without cause for unsatisfactory job performance. Most organizations do not grant new employees the right to appeal a termination decision for failure to satisfactorily complete the probationary period. In these instances, the human resource professional or administrator should review and approve such determinations to ensure that no discrimination has occurred. If an employee files discrimination charges, the employer must defend the action. This is why thorough documentation is essential.

Employment law related to "employment at will" is undergoing significant change currently. Some states have voided the "at will" concept — that an employer may hire or fire at will. Thus, policies about probationary employment should be carefully specified in employee handbooks. For example, if a handbook says "a probationary employee can be discharged at any time during the probationary period," it has been argued that employees who have completed the probationary period are no longer employed at will and are permanent employees. Be sure to check all employment documents to remove any reference to "permanent employee."

For the introductory period to be useful, the job performance of the employee should be evaluated on a regular basis, ideally monthly or at least once every three months. At these times, there should be a discussion with the employee and a written performance evaluation should be completed. If the employee has not progressed satisfactorily, he or she should be notified and terminated any time prior to the end of the introductory period.

Once an employee has successfully completed the "probation" period, the regular performance cycle should be used for planning and evaluation, whether on the anniversary date or at year end, etc. If a performance problem occurs during this period, a new cycle should be established. However, after a few weeks, the employee may still not be performing at the expected standard.

In most cases, the person is given more time to demonstrate improvement. A performance plan should be developed and evaluation should occur within a specified period. Once this period has been successfully concluded, the regular cycle is in effect again. Chapter Eight discusses this cycle in more detail.

Performance interviews

To initiate the PMP with employees, each supervisor should arrange a meeting with each employee. During new employee orientation, employees should be informed by each supervisor about scheduling such a meeting soon. Current staff also should be informed about when their interviews will be scheduled.

When the supervisors schedule the sessions, they should let the employees know what the discussion will cover; i.e., performance evaluation and planning. The employees should be asked to prepare for the session by doing some pre-thinking about topics they would like to cover and by doing some self-assessment of their performance. As mentioned in Chapter Five, using an employee self-evaluation worksheet is recommended.

The interviews should be scheduled as soon after orientation for new employees, and after the introduction of the PMP to current staff, as possible and completed within the first couple of weeks. In this way, employees will feel

Figure 6.3

Supervisors' monitoring checklist

Managers should ensure supervisors are being effective performance managers by asking these questions:

✓ Are the supervisors meeting with employees to plan performance?

✓ Are they regularly observing and documenting significant occurrence of performance, both positive and negative?

✓ Are they providing ongoing feedback, both positive and negative?

✓ Are they catching performance deviations at the start and not letting them balloon into big problems?

✓ Are they encouraging employees to be self-responsible for their performance by reporting on their own progress and on their problems?

✓ Are they dealing with serious performance problems fairly, consistently, directly, immediately and legally?

✓ Are they acting like performance coaches, empowering employees and encouraging them to be all they can be?

✓ Are they walking the talk?

the process is being taken seriously and that they will receive personalized attention.

Performance evaluations

Before meeting with their employees, supervisors should discuss their performance evaluation thoughts and ratings with their managers to obtain agreement. This step ensures that the supervisor has considered all appropriate factors and that the approach is legally defensible. In effect, the manager provides the big picture perspective and ensures that organizational responsibilities related to fair evaluations are met.

It's appropriate at this time for the manager to evaluate the supervisor's behavior related to performance management. A Supervisor's Monitoring Checklist can be used to do this. (See Figure 6.3)

As detailed in Chapter Nine, the interview should cover prior performance — both strengths and weaknesses — by discussing specific examples of performance. Using the forms developed for the PMP, the supervisor and employee discuss performance objectives and factors.

Developmental plans

The interview should also focus on plans for the next performance period. Such plans may relate to specific performance objectives or to general personal development plans, depending on the format chosen.

Personnel decisions

Immediately following the interview, the supervisor should review the results and make any appropriate personnel decisions. These might include promotion, transfer, termination, training or compensation. Such decisions also should be discussed with the supervisor's manager. When a potential problem is anticipated or if the evaluation could lead to some type of disciplinary action, the human resource professional or administrator should be involved to ensure all factors are carefully considered.

The employee should be informed of these decisions at the next meeting when the final copy of the form is discussed, then completed and signed by both parties.

Feedback time

During this summarizing meeting, the supervisor and employee should establish specific times for feedback. Often this becomes an informal agenda item for the weekly or monthly meeting they have. In addition, they should consider either a quarterly or semi-annual formal discussion. Supervisors should never wait until the end of the cycle to share comments about progress. Of course, the supervisor should be giving frequent "one-minute" feedback on a consistent basis, as a coach. And, employees should be encouraged to give and seek feedback as a standard practice. Coaching techniques are discussed in more detail in Chapter Seven.

Process review

Once the PMP has been implemented, it should be reviewed each quarter for the first year. Human resource specialists, managers, supervisors and employees should be surveyed on how it is working. Major problems should be dealt with immediately. Minor problems can be collected and addressed at the end of the year when the entire process should be reviewed and revised, as necessary.

Results monitoring

The key to the system review and the redesign is results. Did the PMP achieve its objectives? Do supervisors find it easy to handle? Do employees feel it is fair? Is it legally defensible? And most important, does it improve communication and performance? Such analysis is critical not only for system effectiveness, but also for supervisor and employee support. If it doesn't work well, no one will believe in it and it will become another "let's pretend" process. The medical practice is then left with little return on its investment and poor morale.

Redesign

It is unlikely that a PMP will be perfect the first time out. It can be expected that "bugs" will be identified in the system — from procedural to semantic. A consistent process review and results monitoring will uncover problems.

Then at year end, the design team should be given the assignment to revise the PMP and update it. Undoubtedly, changes in the organization and in the world will occur that might affect the process. This type of review and appropriate redesign should occur on an annual basis.

Summing up

Implementation of the PMP involves many methodical steps and many people. For smaller groups, using a consultant is recommended who can coordinate and guide the development and implementation of all the tasks/ steps outlined in this book. If each step is carried out thoroughly and thoughtfully and many levels of employees are involved, the initial and ongoing results should be successful. Improvements are always possible and should occur to keep the PMP effective and productive.

Footnotes

[1]*Courtney Price.* The Group Practice Personnel Policies Manual. *Denver, Colo.: Medical Group Management Association, 1991.*

[2]*Courtney Price, Bruce Stickler.* Personnel Postscript. *Summer 1990.*

Tracking progress

Chapter Seven

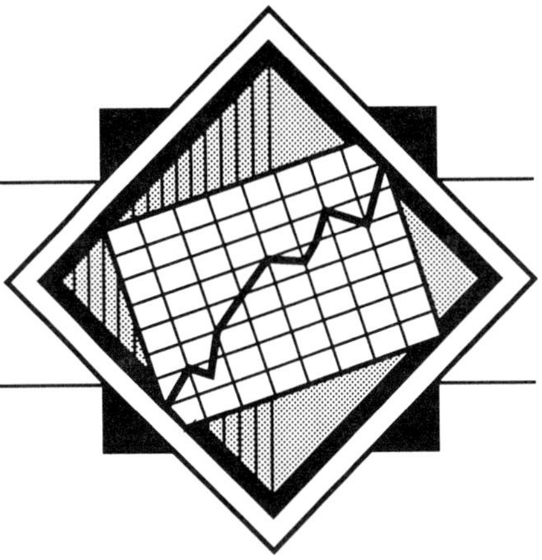

A new supervisor was assigned an employee from another area who management had decided was ready for advancement. The supervisor wasn't sure exactly how to best utilize the employee — and wasn't really sure she wanted her on the team. Over the next few weeks, the supervisor watched the person closely and saw a particular problem that bothered her. She made a long list of incidents when the employee didn't perform the procedure correctly. Then she asked the employee to come in for a discussion. As she proceeded through the list, the employee began to cry. The supervisor stopped and asked, "What is wrong?" The employee replied, "Haven't I done anything right? You are just picking on my Achilles' heel. I know I don't do that procedure very well and I just don't know how to do it better. But I know I do lots of things well."

Ongoing performance discussions between the supervisor and employee are essential and should give the employee balanced feedback on both strengths and weaknesses. However, once the supervisor and employee have discussed performance expectations for the coming performance period, the first true test involves answering these questions:

- Were the expectations clear?
- Were they realistic?
- Were they reasonable in terms of employee ability?
- Were they measurable?

As the journey down the performance path begins, the supervisor should feel like a coach who has worked with the team and developed a game plan. Now, the team must go out on the field and run with the ball — and the coach must stay on the sidelines. Job performance is the job of the performer.

The supervisor's job is to track performance — to observe, to guide via feedback, and if necessary, to diagnose performance problems and to prescribe corrective actions. However, the supervisor is only part of the performance partnership.

The employees have equal responsibility for self-managing their performance. They need to observe their actions and match them against expectations. They should seek feedback regardless of whether the supervisor provides it. They should ask for help with performance problems and participate in developing an improvement plan. Again, supervisors should be key in this effort, coaching employees about taking the initiative. Once employees feel unthreatened, they can admit mistakes and let the supervisor know they don't understand how to deal with a certain situation. They should seek coaching.

The evaluation interview is not the only time to coach. Coaching should take place consistently during the months prior to appraisal. This is possible when performance expectations and measures are clear, and performance problems show up and are solved early. Like effective feedback, coaching for development requires skill, in addition to an appropriately structured situation.

> “When a problem situation has not been addressed soon after it has been identified, it can turn into a horror story. It can get to be a big issue way down the road when it is very hard to turn it around. And it is very difficult for the supervisor to maintain credibility after he/she has let it go on this long. Then we get a conflict of stories with the employee saying, 'I've been doing this for months. Why is it so bad now?'”
>
> *(MGMA member, medium-sized clinic)*

Ongoing progress review

The ongoing progress review involves informing employees on a regular basis about how they are doing in relation to their performance plan. This gives employees important information to help them perform the job more effectively.

If supervisors do not provide employees with this information, there can be a variety of consequences. For example, employees:

- could continue to perform their jobs as they always have, assuming they are doing well;
- may know they are not doing well, but assume that the quality of their work is of no consequence to the supervisor since they get no feedback;
- know if supervisors are not concerned or observing their performance, so they can become careless; and
- may feel unmotivated if they are performing well, and the supervisor fails to notice and give them positive recognition.

Positive feedback

Too often supervisors only give feedback when poor performance occurs. Consequently, the feedback is always negative. However, as Blanchard and Johnson pointed out so effectively in *The One-Minute Manager*, positive feedback is a powerful supervisory tool. Building on concepts that psychologists have long known — reward the performance you want repeated. Blanchard and Johnson promote the use of “one-minute praisings.”[1]

Their model calls for supervisors to:

- praise the positive behavior (with true feelings);
- do it soon after the behavior;
- tell the person what was done right;

- explain how you feel about it;
- encourage the person (with true feelings) to do it again;
- shake hands (or pat the person on the back or make the high sign); and
- proceed with success.

Performance experts suggest that supervisors should use an 80-20 ratio, with 80 percent being positive comments and 20 percent improvement comments. The premise "catch the person doing something right" and reward it has been proven as a very effective technique for reinforcing correct behaviors.

An important point emphasized by David Nadler is that, "Individuals act and organizations function on the basis of information that they receive. People are constantly searching for information to help them make decisions and correct errors, to give them direction and to confirm their beliefs. If information is an important influence on the patterns of behavior of both individuals and organizations, then the use of information may constitute a powerful tool for reinforcing and altering patterns."[2] Thus, feedback of both the positive and negative kinds is extraordinarily useful for supervisors.

Negative feedback

The One-Minute Manager does balance the positive approach with "one-minute reprimands," using a similar model:

- reprimand the behavior (with true feelings);
- do it soon;
- tell the person what was done wrong;
- explain how you feel about it;
- encourage the person (with true feelings);

- shake hands; and
- return to start.

The start for the "One-Minute Manager's Game Plan" is with one-minute goals. In other words, if employees are not clear about their performance objectives and do not perform effectively, it is critical for the supervisor to return to the start. The employee and supervisor should review, clarify and agree on the goals. Then the employee begins again.

If this approach is used consistently, the number of major performance problems should be reduced significantly. Deviations will be caught early and corrected quickly.

Example: Often receptionists are not aware of how important voice tone is when answering patient phone calls. If their voice is flat, the patient may feel that the receptionist not only doesn't care about her job, but also doesn't care about her. This results in a poor impression of the clinic. If the clinic manager does not catch this behavior quickly and provide some feedback, the person will continue unknowingly to erode the clinic's customer service image.

Observation

The essential ingredient for effective feedback is observation. Supervisors can't very well give feedback about something they did not see. The best way to observe, of course, is to be on the scene. Unfortunately, many supervisors in medical practices may not have the luxury of being able to observe their staff on an ongoing basis.

There are several practical methods that help in this situation. One is to dedicate a specific amount of time for observation and coaching when working with a new employee, or with an employee taking on a new task, or with an employee with a performance problem.

The amount of time devoted should depend on the knowledge, skills and abilities of the employee and his or her experience with the organization. A person who is promoted from another position will need little time to learn

> “It is vital to know if your performance management system can deal effectively with problem performers and possible legal situations. We make sure that supervisor feedback is focused on developmental areas so that if there is a performance issue, there will be documentation for progressive discipline. Hopefully, these are identified long before the annual review.”
>
> *(MGMA member, large clinic)*

clinic policies, but will need a certain amount of time to learn a new procedure.

Remember the situational leadership model of tell, sell, coach and delegate introduced in the chapter on supervision. It is not only appropriate but critical for supervisors to tell the new employee what to do and how to do it, then to sell the technique by doing it with him or her, and then watching on the sidelines and coaching the behavior. Rarely can a supervisor walk away and totally delegate performance to an employee, especially a new one.

Cases where this could occur would be with professional staff in a medical practice. In these situations, the manager can rely on a different type of observation — professionals not only must go through rigorous education, they frequently must be certified/licensed on a regular basis.

Their work usually has tangible results that can be observed or is reported (lab reports, patient wound care). In addition, professionals work closely with other professionals who observe their behavior and can serve as coaches.

Managers reach this professional status in another way. They too have gone through rigorous education to reach their positions. They also are closely observed and their actions show up on vital reports such as financial statements, personnel turnover records, or employee grievances.

Observations of workers can be made by other important “audiences” of an employee's performance, as noted previously. These include co-workers, patients and other managers. Information can be obtained through feedback forms such as patient surveys. The information from these groups should be considered carefully. The best observation is the one the supervisor makes himself or herself (and also the one that is legally defensible). However, if there is a pattern of feedback from others about an employee, either positive or negative, the supervisor should pay attention to it and arrange to be on site frequently to observe performance, if possible.

Obviously there will be occasions when the feedback comes after the fact and the moment cannot be recaptured; such as when a patient becomes unhappy about something an employee has or has not done and leaves the clinic in a rage. The supervisor will have to investigate the situation carefully, gather data from the employee and several witnesses, and provide after-the-fact feedback. Then the focus should turn to "how to do it better next time" by asking the employee to develop a plan to avoid the situation in the future.

In the normal tell, sell and coaching stages, the supervisor should assume the role of observer and, like a camera, take snapshots of behavior that can be used as the subject of praises or reprimands. This technique is called the "critical incident" or "significant occurrence" method, as discussed in Chapter Five.

The method involves documenting an occurrence of behavior that is deemed behavior of significant consequence, either positive or negative. Although most traditionally used to document a series of critical incidents that make up a pattern of poor performance, the technique is just as useful for documenting effective performance.

In each case, the documentation is used as a dialog tool with the employee. Typically, a "Critical Incident/Significant Occurrences" form is used that gives the supervisor space in which to describe the incident, the date it occurred, the discussion with the employee about the incident, the corrective action agreed upon (if a negative situation), and both the employee and supervisor sign it.

This document then becomes part of the supervisor's file to be used in performance interviews and to be used for personnel decisions, such as promotion and termination.

The evaluation form can also be used as a note sheet throughout the year to document particularly noteworthy performance by the employee. Many evaluation forms, in fact, include an area for documenting critical incidents during the year.

Critical incidents are anecdotes or brief descriptions of situations in which an employee was particularly effective or ineffective in performing the job. The description might include the circumstances that led to the incident, the consequences of the employee's behavior, or whether the behavior was under the control of the employee. Managers, peers and the employees may enter these descriptions into the performance evaluation records.

The process of recording critical incidents as they occur throughout the year will serve as a memory jogger when the formal evaluation process occurs. Collecting this information consistently throughout the year will result in much greater accuracy in the outcome of the annual evaluation. As noted previously, this information is particularly important in cases where performance is poor enough to warrant disciplinary or termination action.

Some managers meet with their staff monthly to discuss the form and then give a copy to the employee. These forms then become the basis for the annual performance review. This approach eliminates the surprise element in the evaluation process and gives the employee a clear picture of their performance at any time during the cycle.

When giving informal feedback, supervisors should be sure to note what behavior was observed and when on the form. Supervisors should be sensitive to the fact that keeping key performance documentation is for evaluation reasons. They are not keeping a log book on every activity of each employee.

If employees feel they are under constant surveillance in a punitive mode, they will be resentful and their performance will decline. Rather, supervisors should be upfront about documenting significant occurrences — and encourage employees do this too. For example, it is often appropriate to suggest that employees build a "do right" file as well as a "things I have learned" file. It also is appropriate to develop a memo form that employees can use to send their significant occurrence information to their supervisors. This is an excellent technique to get employees involved in managing their own performance.

Observation of performance is a key legal parameter in performance evaluation. For a system to be legally defensible, the evaluation must be done by someone who has regularly observed the employee. That is only fair. Supervisors, therefore, need to practice walk around management, which gives them the opportunity to see behavior on a regular basis.

Sometimes there are situations when a supervisor has been recently promoted to head a work unit and must do evaluations without the opportunity to do much, if any, observation. It is unfair to expect the supervisor to evaluate someone without any data. The answer: The supervisor should get input from others who have been able to observe the employees' performance. This information should be discussed by the supervisor and manager before discussing it with the employees. These steps allow the supervisor to handle this responsibility appropriately.

In all cases, supervisors should always schedule specific times with the employee for more formal observations. They should encourage employees to ask them to sit in, watch them perform and give feedback. For employees who are "in the field," supervisors will need to arrange site visits as well as gather input from the other "audiences," for example, through patient surveys.

The emphasis on observation should be three-fold:

- The supervisor will want to do frequent spot checks to catch the employee in the act and do coaching on the spot.
- The supervisor will want to look for negative patterns that recur and discuss/document them as a means of reinforcing their seriousness about improvement with the employee.
- Employees should be encouraged to observe themselves, to have a built-in mirror that allows them to see the reflection of their behavior.

Performance plan changes

One of the things that supervisors may observe over time is that the performance plan is no longer applicable. This can occur when the supervisor and employee develop a plan with little data; for example, working with a new project where there were lots of unknowns. It can also occur because the work or jobs have changed.

If major shifts in job responsibilities occur, the supervisor and employee should redefine the performance plan, reorder priorities and reassign weights. Unfortunately, in times of restructuring, job responsibilities are often shifted — but performance plans are not modified accordingly.

This is a vital step. The evaluation form used at the end of the performance period must represent as closely as possible the person's real job and therefore should reflect the most current performance plan.

Giving feedback

"Feedback" is part of the two-way communication process. One person sends a message (in words and/or behavior), another person receives it, and returns another message ... feeds back information. (See Figure 7.1)

Figure 7.1

Feedback loop

True two-way communication involves a feedback loop; i.e., supervisor and employee send messages back and forth to ensure each "hears" and understands the other.

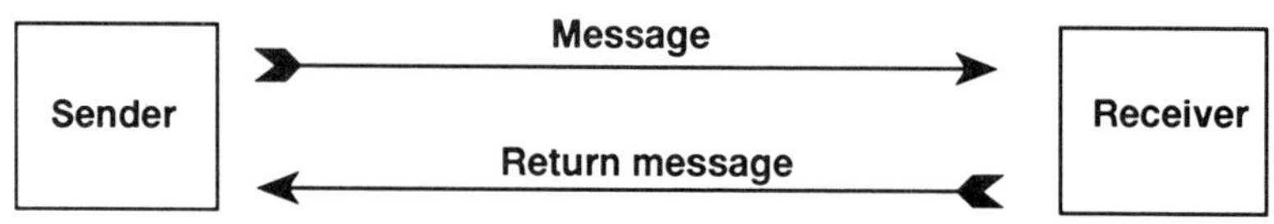

Based on classic communication model.

From a technical view, the problem in providing performance feedback is one of accuracy in measuring performance. In other words, feedback causes problems if it's not grounded in measurement of activities important to the job, if the standards are subjective, or if the appraiser has inaccurate information.

The problem is often compounded by a lack of clearly stated performance expectations. Thus, it is important to anchor the expectations in concrete, observable and measurable terms to begin with, not at the end of the process. Example: Phone calls should be answered by the receptionist within three rings. She should greet the caller with a statement such as "Good morning. This is Pam. How may I help you?" She should smile as she speaks on the phone and modulate her voice to convey enthusiasm.

Reasonably well-defined performance expectations along with specific measurements do not guarantee effective feedback, however. The skills a supervisor uses in saying what needs to be said carry equal importance.

The following principles are recommended by performance management specialist, Marshall Sashkin.[3]

Use descriptive rather than judgmental terms

Judgments block effective communication since they appear to de-value the employee. On the other hand, descriptions of behavior are more acceptable because they are reports rather than value statements.

Judgmental example: "You certainly seem to have a problem with Joe."

Descriptive example: "I was surprised to see you and Joe arguing."

In particular, avoid personal attacks, such as "You are always causing problems."

Be specific and behavioral

Descriptive feedback is most effective when it is specific.

Example: Instead of generally saying, "Your report had two errors," say: "Your report had a typo in line two, and another on line three. I circled them so you can correct them. You are transposing your key strokes."

Remember the receiver's needs

The supervisor and employee have different needs related to feedback. The supervisor wants to help the employee by telling him or her something. The employee may need to hear the information ... but may not want the feedback. In other cases, the employee may seek feedback for psychological/recognition reasons, but may not need it for performance reasons. In both situations, the supervisor should provide feedback, but recognize that the needs of the employee are different.

Give feedback when the receiver is responsive

In general, employees want feedback. However, feedback is only useful when an employee is ready to hear and accept it. Supervisors should be aware that sometimes employees are "not in the mood" for feedback. They should be alert for verbal and nonverbal clues, such as facial expressions and curt responses. Unless the feedback is absolutely essential because of safety or other critical reasons, the feedback should be delayed until the employee is more receptive.

If the "closed ears/mind" mood continues, the supervisor should use some active listening techniques to discover the reason. Example: "You seem uncomfortable about discussing this matter. What is your concern?"

It is vital to choose an appropriate setting for feedback and to offer the employee timing options. This provides a sense of control and encourages participation in moving forward.

Usually the feedback session should occur in a private place. This is always true when negative feedback is given. However, often it is very appropriate to give positive feedback in front of co-workers and others to:

- give some public attention to the person in view of important audiences; and
- to spotlight appropriate behavior for others to emulate.

> "When there is a problem, we give the employee every opportunity to be part of the improvement process and to change the situation. Sometimes you meet with resistance, so this step takes special skill."
>
> *(MGMA member, small clinic)*

Be timely

Immediate feedback is the key to its effectiveness. Individuals learn best by getting a quick response to their behavior. If there is any delay, the specifics of the behavior will be vague and the employee will have difficulty making the connection between the comment and the behavior. There will be situations when the feedback should wait; for example, do not give negative feedback about client relations until after the patient has left. However, usually the faster the comment, the more the employee is likely to understand its significance. This is especially true when the action is negative. Example: When a staff member neglects to follow the correct procedure for handling used syringes, the supervisor must immediately point out the correct, safe way.

Do not ask for the impossible

If an employee does not have control over a situation, there is no point in giving him or her feedback about it. A statement like, "You produce reports too slowly," is unfair when a slow speed printer is all that is available. Instead the focus should be on improving the situation.

Do not attribute hidden motives

In giving feedback, avoid attributing some hidden motive to the other person. Supervisors may have reasons for inferring the motive behind certain behaviors, but these are only guesses and can be easily denied by the employee — and often the guesses are way off track.

Incorrect example: "You are late every day because you really don't like this job," when in reality, the person has a child-care problem.

Correct example: "I am concerned about your lateness. Is there a problem?"

Check to make sure the employee understands the feedback

Miscommunication is the norm rather than the exception. Individuals have selective perceptions and "hear" what they want to hear. To ensure they hear — and understand — the message the supervisor sends, it is useful to have the employee feed it back.

Use a phrase such as: "Tell me what we have agreed to do," or "Would you please review for me your understanding of the situation."

Another method is to ask the employee to write a brief memo or report about the situation or the action plan. Then the supervisor can check to see if it is on target and each person will have a copy to refer to so there are no misunderstandings over time. Documentation is a most useful reinforcer of feedback.

Active listening

Feedback involves both telling and listening. In fact, a very successful way to begin a feedback session is to ask rather than tell, and then listen. Example: "How's it going?" or "What is your opinion?" "How do you see the situation?"

Active listening techniques are helpful at this point, including:

- use body posture and eye contact to show interest (lean forward and look directly at the employee);
- use encouraging words and head nods (uh huh, yeah, yes);

- use inviting, open-ended questions ("How do you feel about that?");

- restate what is said to show real listening and understanding ("You are telling me that the printer is too slow to produce reports as quickly as we need them.");

- check to clarify what was said ("Am I understanding correctly that you are late because the child-care center does not open early enough?");

- sum up, at appropriate points, what was said ("At this point we have agreed that you will investigate other child-care centers and report your findings to me by next week.").

In contrast to these techniques, poor listening is characterized by a telling approach, a "not hearing" response, an impatient attitude. Example: "Tell me what the problem is. I have a couple of minutes right now. I don't care about your child-care problem. You are expected to be here at 8 a.m., or else."

It is useful for supervisors to test their feedback skills by referring frequently to a checklist of key feedback behaviors. (See Figure 7.2 the following page.)

Of particular importance are problems related to avoidance — resistance about giving feedback. Supervisors often feel uncomfortable giving feedback because they "don't want to hurt feelings" or create defensive behavior. A major step for a new supervisor is to realize that not only is giving feedback a vital part of the job, it actually is a "gift" to the employee. By withholding information about poor performance, the supervisor is in effect denying the employee the opportunity to improve before it is too late.

In addition, supervisors should be encouraged to discuss the importance of feedback with employees when developing the performance plan. They should agree on specific times for feedback sessions and on specific tools, like significant occurrence reports and on regular informal feedback on the job.

Another important consideration for supervisors is their own ability to seek and accept feedback. Supervisors should establish the same type of feedback understanding with their own managers, and with their employees.

Figure 7.2

Feedback problem checklist

This list of feedback problems helps supervisors check their effectiveness in giving feedback and gives them clues about skill-building needs.

Avoidance

✓ Avoids giving any feedback
✓ Avoids giving negative feedback
✓ Avoids giving positive feedback

Comparison

✓ Compares one employee against another

Criticism

✓ Attacks the person rather than the behavior
✓ Criticizes several things at once rather than one at a time
✓ Sandwiches negative comments in between positive feedback
✓ Criticizes employees in front of others

Sensitivity

✓ Ignores the employee's receptivity to feedback
✓ Emphasizes own point of view and does not seek employee's
✓ Focuses on proving the supervisor is right rather than finding the cause of the employee's behavior
✓ Uses sarcasm and caustic remarks
✓ Interrupts employee when he/she is responding to the feedback
✓ Gives little consideration to the impact the feedback may have on the future relationship with the employee

Timing

✓ Delays giving feedback until a long time after the incident
✓ Gives feedback when angry, tense or tired

Clarification

✓ Forgets to check to see if the employee "got the message"

Attitude

✓ Feels it is more important to give feedback than to receive it
✓ Feels it is more important to point out mistakes than to problem-solve how to correct them

Method

✓ Prefers to give feedback in writing rather than orally, face-to-face.

Figure 7.3

Ability/motivation matrix

Employees' performance problems should be analyzed in terms of their ability to do the job (can do) and motivation to do the job (will do).

ABILITY: low	ABILITY: high	MOTIVATION
can but won't	can and will	high
can't and won't	can't but will	low

Based on classic motivation theory.

In other words, they should invite their employees to give them feedback too, and then should role model how to accept it undefensively. "Thank you," is always the appropriate response to feedback.

Major performance problems

Occasionally employees will have major performance problems. They will exhibit a pattern of behaviors that is significantly off target and that persists after normal feedback and corrective actions have been taken. This pattern becomes obvious when the "Significant Occurrence/Critical Incident" tracking method is used.

What may not be obvious is why the unsuccessful behavior pattern is occurring. Before proceeding, the supervisor should take the time to determine the cause of the performance problem by considering two key dimensions: motivation (willing) and ability (able).[4]

There are four possible combinations of these dimensions:

- willing and able (not a performance problem);
- willing but unable (an ability problem);
- unwilling but able (a motivation problem); or
- unwilling and unable (both a motivation and ability problem).

When a performance problem is observed as a pattern of continued behaviors and normal corrective feedback has not improved the situation, the supervisor needs to determine which of the three kinds of performance problems are present. (See Figure 7.3)

A model for analyzing performance problems is based on these questions:

- Does the problem involve situational (work context) factors?

- Role definitions and expectations are not clear. Solution: Provide clear specifications of what the worker is responsible for doing and specific task-related coaching assistance.

- Job skills are not adequate. Solution: Provide training assistance.

- Experience is not adequate. Solution: Provide new and different work experiences through appropriate task assignments.

- Degree of involvement in decision making is inappropriate (too little, too great for the individual's ability, or too burdensome). Solution: Adjust the amount of involvement appropriately to gain the correct degree of commitment. Note that sometimes the supervisor's ego gets in the way of participative decision making.

• Is the problem caused by supervisory behaviors?

- Inadequate communication with employees. Solution: Provide the supervisor with skill training in effective listening and giving directions.

- Ineffective feedback skills. Solution: Provide the supervisor with basic skills in giving and receiving feedback to reduce the instances when supervisor's feedback is more likely to do harm than to help the employee improve performance.

- Inappropriate leadership behaviors. Solution: Provide the supervisor with training about situational leadership (learning to vary leadership style according to the dimensions of motivation and ability).

- Ineffective use of rewards. Solution: Provide the supervisor with assistance in how to use cashless compensation/rewards, such as recognition, increased job responsibilities, greater self-control and autonomy, personal praise, and any of the many other non-economic rewards readily accessible to supervisors.

• Is the problem beyond the scope of the supervisor?

- Lack of basic job skills on the part of the employee. Solution: Provide additional formal training or consider a reassignment.

- Personal problems of the employee. Solution: Provide formal counseling via a professional.

In terms of the first type of problem, the supervisor should deal with these on a one-on-one basis with the employee with the focus on improvement of performance and productivity. The process involves the following steps:

Assess the performance situation

How did the unsatisfactory work behavior begin? Attempt to determine the true problem by asking a few key questions such as:

- What has already been tried to solve the problem by the employee, by others?

- What is medical practice policy (if any) about such situations?

- How much ability does the employee have for solving the performance problem?

- Is the employee motivated to help solve the problem?

In all cases, the supervisor should examine the quality of the communication with the employee. The common "I told you" fallacy is based on the false belief that the use of words alone will ensure understanding. The opposite is usually the case. Communication breaks down because the sender fails to understand that his or her meaning is a personal one and may not be the same one held by the one who receives the message.

Define goals

What are the department's goals? What are the goals of the medical practice? Which goals are most pertinent? This is a focusing step to help determine the critical issues and the topics for discussion with the employee.

Generate options

This step represents the possibilities that a supervisor can create to resolve the performance problem. All options should be considered without reservation to get a full sense of what steps can be taken. Some options might include:

- Expect employees to be the best source for generating options since they know the job and themselves best;
- Use outside courses or training programs to build employee's skills;
- Redesign the job to accommodate the employee's skills;
- Create new jobs to spread the work load;
- Spend time coaching employee about performance trouble spots;
- Assign the employee to a senior employee who is a high performer (on-the-job training with a tutor);
- Use co-workers to design a training plan through job rotation; and
- Do goal setting with the employee.

Select a preferred option

In this step, the supervisor should remember that the employee should select the option. The supervisor should serve as "super coach/management problem-solver." In counseling the employee on selecting a performance improvement plan of action, try to examine the risks and benefits of each option — before having the session with the employee. Recognize that the employee not only may have different data about the situation, but also may suggest different options. Be open to these possibilities.

Hold a session with the employee

This step is the most important, since it represents the opportunity to get agreement that there is a problem, to confirm the cause and to develop an improvement plan together. To do this, a technique called "Walk around the Block" is most useful. (See Figure 7.4 on the following page.):

Figure 7.4

Walk-around-the-block performance problem model

Supervisors can use this approach when working with an employee to identify and solve a performance problem. There are four steps:

1. Supervisor identifies a performance problem; discusses it with the employee; employee confirms problem.
2. Employee identifies possible solution; employee and supervisor agree on preferred solution and the number of times it will be tried, and the consequences if not successful; e.g., termination.
3. Employee tries solution for specified period.
4. Supervisor and employee check results at specified time. If satisfactory, the performance improvement is noted in the employee's file. If not, employee tries again for the agreed-upon number of times. If not then successful, the identified consequence occurs.

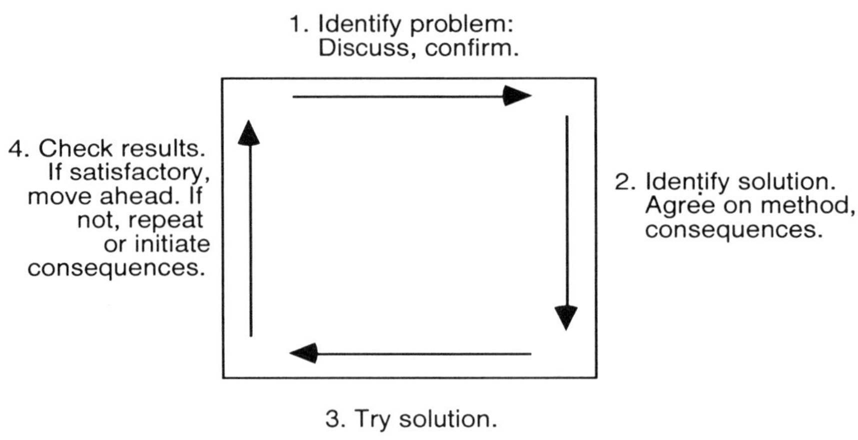

- The supervisor identifies the problem and asks the employee to provide his/her perspective about it. This discussion should continue until there is mutual agreement that there is a problem and it must be addressed.

- The options are discussed and one agreed upon by both the supervisor and employee. The employee's input concerning options is essential. An improvement plan is written and signed by both. Specific actions are noted as well as time and result checkpoints. The amount of leeway in terms of "how many times around the block" is defined. This period may be defined as a probation period, if the problem is a serious one. The consequence of unsatisfactory results is defined; e.g., termination. Feedback dates are established.

- The employee embarks on the improvement plan for the specified period.

- The supervisor and employee have another session on the specified date to discuss results. If the plan has been successful, this is noted on the document and the employee returns to a "regular" status. If results are unsuccessful after the "walks around the block" have been completed, then the agreed upon consequence goes into effect.

This "Walk around the Block" technique is straightforward, easy to document and is legally defensible in terms of giving the employee the chance(s) to improve.

Formal progress reviews

As noted before, mid-year formal reviews are very helpful. However, having quarterly informal progress reviews with each employee is also worthwhile, if possible, or reviews after a major assignment has been completed.

During these progress reviews, the supervisor notes supporting data in the employee's performance evaluation form. Notes, copies of reports, letters of commendation, letters of discipline, activity reports, special projects and any similar items should also be noted on the form and kept in the employee's file. This provides a wealth of information for the final year-end review.

Tracking the employee's performance and giving interim evaluations as projects or major assignments are completed will achieve these results:

- The employee will know the performance management process is for real and the supervisor is serious about expectations.

- The supervisor will have much sounder support to use in the year-end evaluation.

- No one will be surprised at the end of the year. This is one of the biggest problems with performance management. When "surprises" occur, it is clear the performance management system is not working. However, because of the ongoing feedback and the frequent progress reviews built into the recommended PMP, success should be assured. Thus, the evaluation session becomes a time for celebration of a "job well done" and a successful performance partnership.

SUMMING UP

Monitoring performance during the performance period and eliminating the de-motivators that get in the way of performance are two critical tasks for every supervisor. However, that's what management is all about ... the daily focus on getting the highest performance possible by being the coach, the resource that employees can count on to help them be star performers.

FOOTNOTES

[1]*Kenneth Blanchard, Spencer Johnson.* The One-Minute Manager. *New York: Berkley Books, 1981, p. 101.*

[2]*David Nadler.* Feedback and Organization Development: Using Data-Based Methods. *Reading, Mass.: Addison-Wesley Publishing Co., 1977.*

[3]*Marshall Sashkin.* A Manager's Guide to Performance Management. *New York: American Management Association, 1986, p. 21.*

[4]*Patricia King.* Performance Planning & Appraisal. *New York: McGraw-Hill Book Co., 1987, p. 49.*

Legal pitfalls in performance management

Chapter Eight

A medical practice had just hired a new director of nurses, who had very little supervisory experience, but was very knowledgeable about Medicare and other insurance procedures. She inherited a staff that had not had a supervisor for several months. As she began working with the employees, she began to hear more and more complaints about one of the nurses. No one seemed to want to work with her. In turn, that nurse was always complaining about the organization and its procedures. The director had several discussions with the nurse to discuss the situation, but this seemed to make matters worse. When the director discovered that the nurse had complained to the insurance auditors about the way "things are handled here," the director fired the nurse. The nurse promptly filed a suit against the organization, stating that she had a past record of good performance evaluations, had no knowledge that her present performance was "not good enough," had no warning that she was on probation and no opportunity to improve. The medical practice was able to settle out of court — and quickly made sure that the director was brought up to speed about the appropriate steps to take when confronted by a performance problem.

Throughout this manual, there has been constant reference to the need for ensuring that a performance management process is legally defensible. It is a fact of life today that performance evaluation is one of the hottest areas of employment law because it often results in discipline and termination problems.

"Employment-at-will" laws have caused some of these concerns. The traditional concept of an employer's right to hire and fire at will is under attack, with a growing number of states moving toward more employee-oriented legislation. As a result of this focus, suits for wrongful discharge are increasing. In these suits, employees often claim they have received satisfactory performance evaluations for many years before being fired arbitrarily — and some of their concerns are justified.

Example: Organizations that are downsizing occasionally have used the excuse of poor performance to lay off long-time employees. In fact, they want to get rid of those with the highest pay, and the discharge has little to do with performance.

Another reason is a renewed focus on employment discrimination. Current controversies about sexual harassment and the Americans with Disabilities legislation have intensified the spotlight on performance evaluation. Again, if the record fails to show a solid performance-based reason for an employer's action against an individual, claims of discrimination become more credible (such as, hiring bias, barriers to promotion and training, questionable staff reductions, terminations, etc.).

In such situations, if there is little evidence documenting poor performance by employees, the benefit of any doubt almost always goes to the employee. Too often, careless attention to performance planning, ongoing monitoring and frequent evaluation have allowed performance problems to fester without correction, until it's too late for appropriate documentation and improvement. The employee is fired — and the employer fries in the hot seat.

Management pitfalls

Senior managers of medical practices should recognize the numerous ways that can cause legal problems related to performance management. (See Figure 8.1) These include:

- not investing sufficient time, money and effort in developing and maintaining a sound performance process;
- not providing initial and ongoing training about the process for supervisors and written instructions;
- not insisting that the performance process's policies and procedures be used in the actual practice of day-to-day management;
- not ensuring appropriate oversight to spot and correct inadequate supervisory use of the process and serious offenses;
- not requiring that any potential discharge be reviewed by human resource professionals and/or legal counsel before decision and action; and
- not providing override procedures to give employees access to due process methods such as ways to appeal performance evaluations.

Figure 8.1

Legal pitfalls for management

- ➡ insufficient investment in process;
- ➡ insufficient supervisory training;
- ➡ inadequate monitoring of process;
- ➡ inadequate oversight of supervisors;
- ➡ inadequate discharge procedures; and
- ➡ inadequate due process procedures.

Supervisory pitfalls

In addition to management oversight, supervisors should avoid these problem areas (See Figure 8.2 on the following page.):

- giving little to no attention to upfront performance planning;
- providing inadequate feedback during the performance period;
- failing to do ongoing performance observation as a means of spotting performance problems and correcting them immediately;

Figure 8.2

Legal pitfalls for supervisors

- inadequate performance planning;
- inadequate feedback;
- inadequate performance observation;
- inadequate attention to performance interviews;
- neglect or delay of evaluations;
- not honest, not thorough;
- giving "average" ratings;
- giving "inflated" ratings;
- wanting to be "nice";
- being biased;
- being too friendly; and
- not being serious about performance management.

- spending little time on completing performance forms and holding performance interviews;
- neglecting to do regular evaluations, or delaying them for long periods of time;
- not being honest and thorough;
- giving staff an "average" rating because no actual data about performance was collected since "it takes too much time";
- giving "inflated" ratings that cover up mediocre performance or legitimate faults because of guilt over not dealing with them;
- wanting to be the "nice person" who is well-liked;
- being subjectively biased about certain employees and making judgments without regard to job-related criteria;
- being too friendly with employees and thus being unable to evaluate performance objectively; and
- not taking performance management seriously.

Process credibility

The only way to avoid such pitfalls and to prevent claims and suits is to have a credible system and supervisors who are well trained in its use. No medical practice can afford to be vulnerable to litigation because it has failed to establish:

- job-related, behaviorally oriented performance standards that are communicated effectively to employees;
- an accurate, detailed record of the employee's performance; and
- supervisors who understand that managing the performance of employees is the key to their own successful performance.

Performance documentation has always been necessary for formal grievance procedures. It is also necessary before an employee can be discharged. There must be an accurate record that shows the specific problems and the efforts made to improve them.

There also needs to be a system for catching any sudden switches in a supervisor's evaluation. For instance, management should be concerned when an employee who has had a series of favorable evaluations suddenly becomes a performance problem. It is fairly rare for a good performer to develop performance problems over night. More likely, the supervisor has failed to document a consistent problem or is now judging the person more negatively for another reason, such as a personality conflict.

It is vital that supervisors understand the prime reason for performance management. An effective performance management process is not just legal protection. It provides significant management leverage. Effectively used, the process enhances motivation and productivity. Consistent, objective evaluation of the employee's performance, that is based on measures of actual performance according to standards directly related to the job, provides information about: the employee's current performance, his or her potential for development, performance problems to be corrected, training/experience needed. Such data provides the basis for compensation, succession, development, or termination decisions.

Performance management processes are particularly useful for identifying training needs. Evaluations can help supervisors determine if there is an appropriate match between the employee's skills and the job's requirements. If there is a gap, the supervisor then can provide appropriate training. Correcting any mismatch via training can raise morale, provide new incentives for productivity and reduce turnover and termination.

If termination is the chosen course of action, by carefully documenting the employee's performance shortfalls, giving the person fair notice of the problems and giving him or her several chances to improve, the employer establishes a solid factual basis for discharge. Records of specific incidents and behaviors, as well as documentation of efforts to work with the employee to improve performance, demonstrate there is good cause for termination and provide the basis for a solid court case.

In turn, an inadequate method based on knee-jerk reactions and poorly documented judgments is a major risk, with high potential for setting off legal bombfires that could be very costly in time, money and morale. If a medical practice cannot prove it has a fair, impartial performance process, it is a sitting duck just waiting for a big gun to shoot it out of the water.

Legal basis

There is much law today that directly ties performance evaluation with the legal system. Many laws and court rulings since the 1960s have included either explicit or implied sections that require employers to document employee performance before making various human resource decisions. These laws, along with strong government pressure in these areas and increased litigation, have motivated organizations to implement formal, systematic performance evaluation processes.

Some of the most important laws are:[1]

- The Civil Rights Act of 1964 (and as amended in 1972) and Equal Employment Opportunity Commission guidelines were the initial impetus for this change because of their focus on all personnel decisions, including performance evaluation. These laws, which ban employment discrimination, require fairness in employment procedures and valid procedures for appraising performance. For example, the 1978 Uniform Guidelines on Selection Procedures state that the job-relatedness of "selection devices" such as performance evaluation must be demonstrated by validation; i.e., relevance.

  It is critical for medical practice managers to understand that any procedure, formal or informal, scored or unscored, which is used to make any personnel decision, including hiring, promotion, transfer or dismissal is covered by these federal guidelines. This includes performance evaluations, which are considered to be "tests" under these laws.

  These laws protect all American citizens. The laws specifically state that an employer may not discriminate on the basis of race, religion, sex or national

❝We are close to a legal problem now. We have a situation where an employee's job grew without changes being made in her job description, and indeed without authorization. It just sort of happened. The situation has become a monster. The person was not a great performer to begin with. All of this happened because of good intentions. We just got sucked in because we didn't lay out expectations and set parameters. The job description went askew. It probably means the person will be hurt because the situation has to change — and if we let her go, we may be in trouble.❞

(MGMA member, rural, small clinic)

origin. Because of past discrimination, attention was initially focused on the protection of racial minorities and females. Now increased emphasis is being placed on the protection of older individuals and people with disabilities.

The government agencies who are responsible for insuring compliance with the law are the Equal Employment Opportunity Commission, the Office of Federal Contract Compliance, the Department of Labor, the Department of Justice and federal courts.

- The Equal Pay Act of 1963, which states that men and women whose jobs require equal skill, effort and responsibility should also receive equal pay.
- Executive Orders 11246 and 11375 of 1965 and 1967, which prohibit discrimination by federal agencies and contractors and call for affirmative action programs when women and minorities are under-represented in their job categories.
- The Age Discrimination in Employment Act of 1967, which states that all employees must be treated fairly, regardless of age.
- The Rehabilitation Act of 1973, which bans employers who receive federal funds from discriminating against people with disabilities.
- The Pregnancy Discrimination Act of 1978, which put expectant mothers under the protection of the Civil Rights Act.
- The Americans with Disabilities Act of 1990, which promotes both accessibility and employability for people with disabilities.
- The Family Leave Act of 1993, which requires organizations with more than 50 employees to allow 12 weeks of unpaid leave because of an employee's illness or that of a parent, spouse or dependent child. In addition, when the person returns, he or she must be reinstated to his or her current or similar job with no loss of status.

Validity and reliability

It is advisable to validate all personnel decision-making procedures, including the performance management process. However, validation is required only if there is adverse impact on individuals or groups protected by Title VII of the Civil Rights Act. The law does not state that this step must be taken when developing the system; however, if the procedures are ever questioned, the employer must prove they are valid.[2]

Employers who do not want to validate their procedures (or cannot, for financial or other reasons) can adjust employment procedures to eliminate potentially discriminating conditions. For example, they can hire and promote employees using procedures, such as random selection, that ensure a representative proportion of minorities and women in relevant jobs.

This option sometimes means making employment decisions based on criteria other than merit, which can be counterproductive to an employer's need for performance and productivity. These options also tend to be counterproductive in that they are often labeled reverse discrimination.

Proof of validity of a procedure must be based on empirical data, not just a professional's opinion. That is, employers must prove that any procedure, such as a performance evaluation tool, measures what it is supposed to measure, or it is not valid.

To demonstrate the validity of a procedure, an employer must show that the behaviors described in the evaluation tool represent the content of the job. The closer the content is to work samples or work behaviors, the stronger is the basis for showing content validity.[3]

This is a pragmatic or logic-based validity. It requires an easily identifiable relationship between evaluation form items and job-related activities, situations and outputs. It is an apples-to-apples comparison method.

A simple example: An appropriate measure of typing ability is a typing test that measures accuracy and speed. A criterion based on years of education would be inappropriate since it has no relevance to the ability to type.

Performance evaluations also must be reliable. Reliability is a measure of the consistency or stability of a test or other measure over time and with its use by different raters. A reliable test is one that provides similar or comparable results regardless of when it is used or who uses it.

Feedback is also a critical part of a legally defensible performance management process. Employees who have performed poorly must be informed of their deficiencies and have the opportunity to request additional training and experience, and then to be re-evaluated. Thus, employers must pay increased attention to the issues of feedback and the right to information.

Compliance

Suggestions for complying with the law include:

- Employers should have records of job applicants, new employees and promoted and demoted employees categorized by race, sex, national origin, religion, age, disability. Although this step is most important in terms of job applicants, it is also useful data for all human resource decisions. These records will document whether or not the proportions of applicants/ employees are considerably different from those in the population of the community. As a standard operating procedure, medical practice managers should review such data regularly.

- Employers should have a formal evaluation system. An informal system cannot be validated. Employers with no formal process would be found liable in any case where *prima facie* evidence of discrimination exists. Employers must be able to demonstrate that their employment practices are based on job-related criteria and not on any prejudicial intent. A formal evaluation system is the proof.

The courts do acknowledge the employer's right to evaluate employees' on-the-job performance. The guidelines are aimed to prevent evaluation systems that are not designed appropriately, are not based on job-related criteria and are not applied consistently and fairly.

The key to a legally defensible process: the use of actual job performance measures — whenever possible. Supervisory ratings of job performance are subject to suspicion. These ratings are considered less reliable because of the possibility of subjectivity. The premise: Rater bias may result in negative evaluations of protected groups.

In sum, the key legal requirements are:

- There should be a direct link between job requirements and performance measurement tools.
- High scores should reflect high job performance.
- The procedure should be a reliable predictor of future performance.
- The tools should provide a valid measure of the employee's motivation and intelligence/ability.

Right to privacy

Another legal aspect to keep in mind is right to privacy. More and more states have statutes that protect employees' access to their files.[4]

Specifically, employees whose data are collected must have access to their data and must have the opportunity to challenge and correct it. In regard to access, it is important to realize that during a person's employment with the medical practice, employees have the right to have copies of their performance evaluations. After each review and after both parties have signed the form, the employee should get a reference copy; the supervisor should keep a copy; and/or put a copy in the personnel file. The employee should have access to that file. Those with legitimate access are the supervisor, management and the human resource staff. Others should not have access. This policy should be covered in the medical practice's policies and procedures manual.

After employees have left the organization, generally they have no legal right to obtain their performance records. These documents are considered to have been prepared for corporate purposes using company resources, and therefore, belong to the organization. This issue sometimes comes into play when a person is seeking such records to use as reference information. Because of the increasing number of defamation suits related to giving references, many organizations now follow a "no reference" policy.[5]

Good faith requirement

Medical practice managers must recognize that there is an implied requirement of good faith and fair dealing in the employment relationship. The good faith requirement comes into play whenever an employer makes "objective manifestations that lead an employee to believe he or she has job security and will be treated fairly." Such demonstrations include promotions and a series of favorable performance evaluations.

The good faith requirement seeks to balance possible unequal bargaining positions. Employees should not be expected to bend over backwards to satisfy the employer just to avoid termination.[6]

Wrongful discharge

More and more often workers who have been terminated are going to court claiming "wrongful discharge" and more frequently courts are agreeing. The premise: Employees have the right to be treated fairly in discharge situations.

"Fairly" is defined in two ways. One: ensuring that employees have been objectively and impartially evaluated via a sound performance evaluation process. Two: ensuring that employers do not arbitrarily dismiss employees with a history of satisfactory evaluations.

As noted before, the increase in wrongful discharge suits is a direct challenge to the tradition of employment-at-will — a tradition unique to the United States. It means that either the employer or employee can end the employment relationship at any time for any, or no, reason. No other country allows such unrestricted freedom of choice by either party.[7]

Actually, this concept is a relatively new idea — only about 100 years old. Previously, it was assumed that employment was for a definite period agreed on in advance by two parties who were then bound by the arrangement; such as an apprenticeship. Thus, the idea of employment-at-will (an employee can be discharged for any or no reason) was seen as a step forward, particularly for employers.

It still exists, but more frequently today there are demands for basing a discharge on a legitimate reason. One long-time exception to the tradition is the public policy exception. In this case, the law and established public policies are judged to be more important than an employer's interest.

Another exception relates to employment contracts that promise, in effect, that employees can keep their jobs as long as their work is satisfactory. Although few employees have written work contracts, many employee handbooks and personnel policy manuals state that an employee can only be discharged for "good cause" and the courts say this statement constitutes a contract.

For this reason, employment lawyers advise that a statement about "employment-at-will" be included in application forms and personnel manuals with a statement that the offer of employment or manual does not constitute an employment contract. Words like "permanent employee" also are no longer used. In addition, employers are reminded that an oral promise of job security is as binding as a written one.

A related issue is that of a "covenant of good faith." Some courts now hold that an employment "bargain" between an employer and employee occurs when there is a long work history. The premise: During an extended period of service, the employer develops an obligation to the employee, a duty not to take away the job without giving a valid reason. A promise of job security is implied and it cannot be broken without a legitimate reason.

Judges and juries are particularly sympathetic to a long-term employee. The longer the term of service, the more good faith is expected. This premise particularly covers the long-term employee whose skills are becoming obsolete. An effort to provide training or another position is a demonstration of good faith.

If an employee is terminated in such a case, the courts will be favorably impressed if the medical practice has acted courteously and compassionately. That is, if the records prove that the employer took special care to give the person adequate notice and outplacement assistance after training and other internal job opportunities proved unfeasible, few juries, judges or hearing officers will find that the organization acted in bad faith.

Another exception to employment-at-will is the case of undue emotional distress. Intentionally subjecting an employee to such distress is held to be going beyond "all possible bounds of decency." Example: imposing impossible deadlines.[8]

A case of wrongful discharge is very likely to be upheld if an employer has demonstrated extreme and outrageous conduct. Example: An employee is given a poor evaluation in retaliation for filing a grievance. Every evaluation should accurately and impartially reflect the employee's actual performance.

AGE DISCRIMINATION

A growing area of litigation relates to age discrimination. This is another reason for a sound, performance-based evaluation process. If a medical practice is sued for age discrimination, the case could be won or lost on the basis of its process.

The Federal Age Discrimination in Employment Act covers hiring, firing, promotion, demotion, discharges, transfers and changes in existing jobs. It protects employees over 40 years old against discrimination in these employment actions.

There are three major defenses against an age discrimination suit:

- Establishing that age is a bona fide occupational qualification. That is, there is a legitimate reason for not hiring a person over 40 years of age for the job. Simple example: hiring a child to play the hero's role in the movie "Home Alone," rather than a 60-year-old person. Another example: terminating airline pilots

> "We keep seeing 10-page evaluations from supervisors that are dialogs about employees that walk on water. This happens even though others observe the employees coming in late, not carrying their share of the work load, complaining and grumbling. The evaluations say nothing about quality, accuracy, etc. If we have to terminate these employees, we will have no documentation to back up our position."
>
> *(MGMA member, large clinic)*

when they reach 60 years of age because research to date indicates decline of physical abilities at that age;

- Establishing that there is a bona fide seniority or merit system. In this case, there must be a consistent pattern of personnel decisions based on length of service or meritorious performance. Merit, of course, can only be proven by a solid performance management process; and

- Establishing that a Reasonable Factor Other Than Age (RFOTA) is the reason for the personnel decision. In other words, a medical practice needs to be able to prove it had a reason other than age to take a certain personnel action (selection, promotion, termination). Example: A group practice decides for business reasons that it no longer will offer a certain service and that decision affects an older person who has been providing that service.

There are two basic requirements to establish an RFOTA:

- Establishing fair, nondiscriminatory standards for judging all employees; measuring the employee against specific standards. More subjective criteria, such as a supervisor's general impressions of an employee's ability to work, are not considered sufficient; and

- Applying these standards in a consistent, visible manner (regularly conducting performance planning and evaluation interviews with all employees as an ongoing standard operating procedure).[9]

In cases of age discrimination, as well as others, courts are adverse to after-the-fact evaluations. Evaluations that appear to have been developed after a negative personnel decision are looked at with a very critical eye.

Another pitfall: Unreasonable workloads given to an older employee, who then receives a poor evaluation. This is likely to be perceived as a conscious effort to force failure.

As always, a pattern of consistent, regular, valid evaluations is the best defense in cases of age discrimination.

Sexual and racial discrimination

The rules related to sexual and racial discrimination are similar to those used for age; that is, a fair process not influenced by discriminatory factors. However, there is one important difference. Race/sex discrimination laws are equally concerned with the impact of employers' well-intended acts as they are with deliberate discrimination.[10]

Example: In the past, tests were used with good intentions to select employees on the basis of ability. However, many tests turned out to have adverse impact because they used the language of the dominant culture, and thus discriminated against people of another culture.

In these cases, a performance management process and decisions based on that process are satisfactory demonstrations that personnel decisions are not discriminatory. Once again, the key to success is a process that is specifically job related.

As always, the best defense to a claim of racial or sexual discrimination is a process directly tied to job requirements based on thorough and regular job analysis, and current job descriptions. The evaluation process must be built on solid performance standards. Most important, employees must be informed of the standards by which they will be judged.

There is another sex discrimination factor to keep in mind. The Equal Pay Act requires that men and women whose jobs are equal in terms of the compensable factors of skill, effort, responsibility and working conditions must receive equal pay, with one exception. A bona fide seniority or merit pay system can justify pay differentials. That is, if a medical practice has a long record of paying employees on the basis of tenure and men happen to have the longest tenure, then it is acceptable to pay them more.

It is also acceptable to pay a man more if his performance is better than a woman's in the same job. Again, a solid performance process must be used to support a merit pay system. That is, performance ratings must be used to set pay rates when a merit system is used. Such ratings are "sex-less."

Recent employment cases have put new emphasis on the link between sexual harassment and performance evaluation (harassment and retaliation for an employee's complaints often result in low evaluations).

The EEOC's "Guidelines on Sex Discrimination" state that "unwelcome sexual advances ... have the purpose or the effect of unreasonably interfering with an individual's work performance or creating an intimidating, hostile or offensive working environment." In sum, an employer is responsible for indirect as well as direct effects of harassment and resulting poor performance.[11]

Sexual discrimination can occur in parenting cases as well. Employers can come to suspect conclusions about the effects of pregnancy and motherhood on performance. In addition to making assumptions about the ability of a woman to perform in these situations, supervisors may have subjective personal beliefs about the "rightness" of a pregnant woman or mother working.

The courts find that personnel decisions made on assumptions or personal reactions are not valid. Only those based on factual, documented performance records are admissible.

Tips for a defensible system

The following recommendations will help medical practices ensure the defensibility of their performance management systems:

- Have a formal, standardized, objective process;
- Base the process on clear, specific, communicated job requirements and expectations;
- Conduct formal, thorough job analyses for all positions on a regular basis (at least every two years and more frequently if the job changes);
- Insure against the potential for subjective supervisory ratings by making them just one part of the process;

- Train evaluators thoroughly about the proper use of the process;
- Insist that those who evaluate the employee have frequent opportunities to observe his or her performance;
- Insure a higher degree of objectivity by having more than one evaluator;
- Standardize the administration and scoring of the evaluation tool;
- Post promotion/transfer opportunities;
- Allow employees to initiate promotions/transfers without his or her immediate supervisor's recommendations;
- Document reasons for all employment decisions;
- Use performance criteria that do not adversely impact protected groups;
- Provide evaluation forms and instructions on their use to all evaluators;
- Keep employee records private and allow only the individual, the supervisor, senior management and the human resource specialist to have access to the records; and
- Put procedures ensuring due process into effect and observe them consistently.

Ethics and due process

There is a fundamental belief that underlies a performance management process. "Workplace ethics require that people be judged solely on the basis of job performance." It is unethical to judge the person rather than the performance.[12]

In addition to today's focus on business ethics, employers should also recognize the trend toward increasing due process rights — employees are due (owed) fair treatment.

This is part of the implied "contract" based on the exchange of value that occurs when a medical practice provides rewards/compensation for an employee's performance/work.

A program that offers due process opportunities to employees includes these steps:

- telling new employees about the performance management process — what it is and how it works;
- explaining expectations and providing appropriate training;
- working with employees to develop performance plans, standards and objectives;
- expecting and encouraging employees to do self-assessments of their own performance;
- encouraging employees to ask for and to give feedback; and
- rewarding behaviors that fulfill performance expectations.

In addition, a due process program ensures that the medical practice follows these procedures:

- a higher level management review of a supervisor's evaluations;
- a human resource specialist monitoring of the supervisor's evaluations and performance management behaviors;
- management commitment to regular auditing of the performance management process; and
- management provision for an appeals process to deal appropriately and fairly with grievances.

Figure 8.3

Due process premises

1. Body of rules
2. Right to voice case
3. Fact-based decisions, burden of proof on all parties
4. Everyone treated the same

The essence of due process rests in the right to appeal. The appeals process is based on these premises (See Figure 8.3):

- a body of rules that everyone agrees to follow;

- the right of each person to state his or her case;
- decisions made on the basis of fact with the burden of proof the responsibility of all parties; and
- an effort to treat everyone the same.

In sum, a fair process will be: visible, predictable, institutionalized, equitable, easy to use and applicable to all employees.

Summing up

Incorporating the following elements into the medical practice's performance management process should increase the likelihood that the process will withstand legal scrutiny, if challenged:

- current job description;
- job-related criteria;
- specific, realistic performance standards;
- ongoing feedback;
- performance counseling/training/development opportunities;
- formal training for supervisors on the entire process;
- written instructions on the performance evaluation form;
- evaluation results reviewed with employees;
- review/audit/appeal procedures in place; and
- documentation/records.

Most of all, medical practices should remember that although having a performance management system that is legally defensible is critical, the most important reason for a sound system is as a positive tool to improve organizational and employee/individual performance.

FOOTNOTES

[1]*J. Vernon Odom, Keith J. Edwards.* Performance Appraisal: Legal Aspects. *Greensboro, N.C.: Center for Creative Leadership, 1977, p. 108.*

[2]*Beatty, p. 47.*

[3]*Odom, p. 110.*

[4]*ibid, p. 113.*

[5]Business and Ethics. *"Employees Deserve a Look at Their Files,"* Rocky Mountain News, *July 22, 1992, p. 52.*

[6]Performance Appraisals: The Latest Legal Nightmare. *Maywood, Ind.: Modern Business Reports, 1989, p. 10.*

[7]*ibid, p. 20.*

[8]*ibid, p. 22.*

[9]*ibid, p. 46.*

[10]*ibid, p. 62.*

[11]*ibid, p. 82.*

[12]*Charles R. McConnell.* The Health Care Manager's Guide to Performance Appraisal. *Gaithersburg, M.D.: Aspen Publishers, 1993, p. 207.*

The performance interview

Chapter Nine

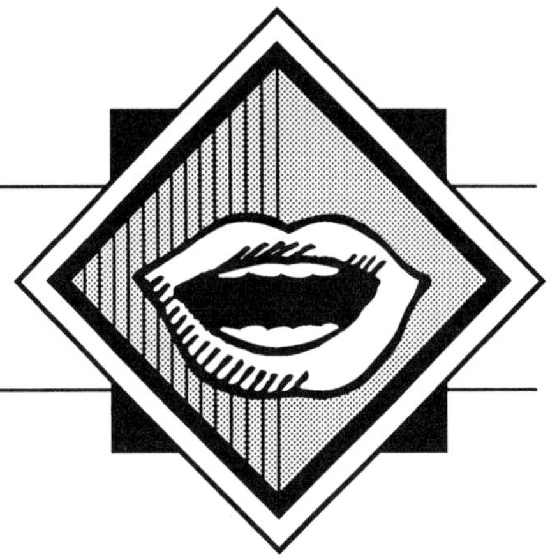

A supervisor in a small medical practice prided himself on the fact that he completed the performance reviews for all seven employees who reported to him in less than a day. He spent the morning filling out the forms and then called each employee into his office and read him or her the evaluation. It was very straightforward and very efficient. It usually took less than 15 minutes each — unless an employee had some questions, which typically related to raises. At the end of the day, the supervisor marked the task as "done till next year." Or was he? Very often there were occasions during the year when employees didn't seem to know what was expected. Then he had to spend hours and hours walking through what he thought "everyone knew." And, the employees he thought should show improvement never seemed to move out of status quo.

The performance cycle is uniquely tied to its finale — the annual performance interview. Throughout the performance period, the supervisor hopefully has been giving feedback to the employee. However, the final session, which actually is a performance review/preview and signifies the end of one performance period and the beginning of the next, is very special.

> “The best kind of performance interview is a situation where the supervisor and subordinate meet two to three times a year and give equal input about what the subordinate's needs are and how well the subordinate is doing. This type of conference shows that there is a performance partnership.”
>
> *(MGMA member, medium-sized clinic)*

It has symbolic importance because it marks a significant milestone, a time when supervisor and employee meet to discuss how they did together in their performance partnership. This session is often held in conjunction with the employee's anniversary date. This is useful symbolism to reinforce the concept of mutual commitment that pays off for both partners.

If the partners have done well during the year, the session should be a celebration of “how well we've done.” There will be no surprises because the supervisor and employee have been together throughout all the twists and turns of the year. They have agreed on corrections in behaviors, modified performance plans to reflect changes encountered along the way and conferred frequently to ensure performance was on the success track.

If there had been a major performance problem, it had been dealt with immediately using the “Walk around the Block” method of problem-solving, action planning and making the effort to improve.

Nine out of 10 times this process will have worked successfully and the employee is off probation and back on track. If the probation/discipline process was not successful, the consequences have been exercised and the employee is no longer with the medical practice.

Therefore, the focus of performance interviews is on working with the competent employee to review what has been learned in the past year and to preview what should be accomplished in the new year. Indeed, it is worthwhile to utilize this session like a New Year's Day to reflect backwards and to project forwards. This focus is both professional and personal since one of the vital parts of the performance interview is its spotlight on personal development.

OBJECTIVES OF THE ANNUAL PERFORMANCE INTERVIEW

The specific objectives for this annual session are to (See Figure 9.1):

- acknowledge an employee's right to know his or her performance is evaluated as a whole body of work by the supervisor at least once a year;
- provide data to management that will be used to make future decisions about job assignments and compensation;
- create a positive climate for constructive dialog to ensure an ongoing productive relationship between the employee, the supervisor and the organization;
- increase the overall productivity level of the organization through an emphasis on specific performance objectives and continued growth of the individual; and
- improve the employee's performance — the bottom line of the performance management process.

Figure 9.1

Performance interview objectives

Supervisors should achieve five objectives during the annual performance interview:

❶ Assess performance data as a total package;

❷ Gather data for future human resource uses;

❸ Maintain a positive relationship with the employee;

❹ Increase potential for organizational productivity; and

❺ Pinpoint areas of employee improvement.

To achieve these objectives, the performance interview should be considered as just one part of the total performance management process — not the end all and be all. Before jumping into the interview session, it is useful to review the entire process in order to put the interview into perspective.

REMEMBERING THE CYCLE

The performance-reward cycle (See Figure 9.2 on the following page) began with the development of a performance plan for the year. This session between the supervisor and employee allowed the supervisor to reiterate the organization's philosophy and policies related to performance management. Also during this session the supervisor and employee reached a mutual understanding of performance criteria and related standards.

Figure 9.2

Performance-reward cycle

Supervisors should remember that employees will perform satisfactorily to meet organizational goals when the rewards they receive fulfill their own needs.

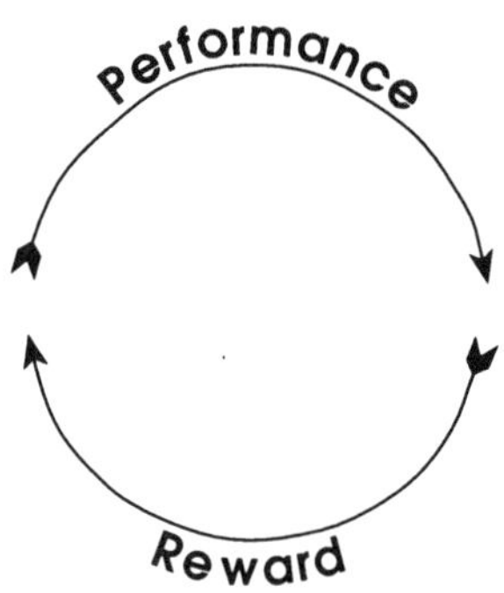

The supervisor reinforced the concept of ongoing communication during the performance period to ensure there is accurate feedback to produce changes in behavior and improved productivity. Performance expectations were discussed in detail so there was no misunderstanding about the basis for evaluation.

This session also included an opportunity for the employee to share his or her self-assessment. The supervisor invited the employee to evaluate himself or herself in terms of strengths, needs for improvement and career goals. These factors were built into the performance plan — new responsibilities were assigned, additional training was scheduled, career counseling resources were identified.

At this time, the supervisor and employee also agreed upon a schedule for ongoing, informal discussions about performance. This might have been during regular meetings, specific monthly or quarterly reviews, or a formal mid-year review, as well as the year-end interview. Whatever the schedule, the critical focus was on commitment to a never-ending dialog about what is and should be happening in terms of performance objectives.

In particular, the supervisor emphasized that the employee is equally responsible for giving and seeking feedback during the year. If the employee had trouble with a certain objective, if he or she discovered a better way to achieve the same goal, if the job changed, if the supervisor was not being as helpful as needed, then the employee had the responsibility — and the right — to speak up.

The supervisor committed to encouraging this initiative by frequently asking the employee for such feedback and receiving it in a welcoming fashion. The supervisor observed the employees closely and frequently during the period, kept notes on the employee's performance and shared these with the employee.

PREPARING FOR THE INTERVIEW

Assuming that the performance-planning launch and the follow through were successful, the supervisor can glide into the interview session with confidence and comfort. The interview is designed as a face-to-face meeting between the supervisor and employee for the primary purpose of exchanging information and ideas. Neither party should actually conduct the interview; both need to experience it.

However, even with a successful year behind them, the interview can be a complex, emotional interaction for both the supervisor and employee. It has the potential for generating perceptual differences, defensiveness, conflict and hostility as a result of faulty listening and misunderstandings. Result: Often what should be a positive learning opportunity and a step forward turns into a wounding experience for both people.

In order to ensure both a constructive and positive session, the performance interview must be conducted in a manner that does not damage the employee's self-esteem. He or she has a right and an obligation to participate equally in the discussion. The employee also has the right to be treated fairly and with dignity and courtesy.

A constructive discussion can be achieved by following these steps:

- Both parties should prepare for the discussion. The individual, as well as the supervisor, should think about the review in advance. Both should make notes about the areas to be covered in the discussion on the appropriate PMP forms about such topics as:
    - how well expectations and objectives were achieved;
    - what problem areas and concerns have arisen and why;
    - how the employee's contributions could be enhanced;
    - what plans for development should be considered; and
    - what goals should be set for the future;
- The traditional authoritarian, parental nature of the interaction should be avoided by:

> "We want to build ownership into job performance. We want to train supervisors to get specific about behaviors that actually occurred — to look at the behaviors and to coach employees during performance reviews. Example: When a patient called, I overheard your response and the perception I got was that you didn't care about the customer. You said, 'We don't do that. We can't help you.' And then you hung up. I am sure that it wasn't a matter of caring — but it came across that way. What might have been a better way to deal with that patient?"
>
> *(MGMA member, large clinic)*

- conducting the interview in a neutral site, such as a conference room rather than in the supervisor's office; and
- structuring the discussion in such a way that both individuals participate as equals. Ensure two-way communication by giving the initiative to the employee. Discuss the employee's topics, concerns, and ideas before the supervisor's viewpoint is presented. Maintain a problem-solving approach. The focus should be on future opportunities and plans rather than on past failures.

Rating errors

Before beginning the performance interview process, supervisors should stop and remember the human fallacies that can adversely impact performance evaluations. Rating errors can occur because of built-in biases that are often unconscious.

The following are ways to provide protection against these prejudices:

- Build safeguards into the performance management process; namely, by building a process that is objective and behavioral and thus less susceptible to subjectivity;
- Use multiple reviewers, when appropriate, so that one person's perspective is balanced by others;
- Ensure that supervisors' reviews are reviewed by their managers as a check against a pattern of bias;
- Remind supervisors of the 50 percent rule; i.e., supervisors should talk less than 50 percent of the time during a performance review. Ideally, they should talk only 20 percent to 30 percent of the time so that the employee has plenty of time to discuss what's important to him or her; and
- Introduce supervisors to classic rating errors during the initial training about the system, and then reinforce this topic during subsequent training on performance management.

The classic rating error list includes (See Figure 9.3):

- halo effect (rating an employee excellent on one factor and then giving a higher-than-deserved rating on other factors);
- horn effect (rating an employee unsatisfactory on one factor and then giving a lower-than-deserved rating on other factors);
- central tendency (rating all factors as average);
- strict rating (rating consistently lower than the expected norm);
- lenient rating (rating consistently higher than the expected norm);
- latest behavior (rating influenced by the most recent behavior rather than behaviors over time);
- performance dimension order (rating one factor like another because they are in close proximity on rating form);
- initial impression (rating based on first impressions rather than behavior over time);
- spillover (rating based on past performance appraisals);
- status effect (over-rating employees in higher-level jobs or jobs held in high esteem or vice versa);
- same as me (rating higher than deserved because employee has qualities like the rater);
- different from me (rating lower than deserved because employee is unlike rater);
- stigma (rating based on the non-acceptance by co-workers of the employee); and
- future use (rating based on some perceived future use of the appraisal).

Supervisors should review this error list each time they are preparing for a performance interview.

Figure 9.3

Rating error checklist

Supervisors can fall prey to making these errors when evaluating an employee:

- ✔ halo effect;
- ✔ horn effect;
- ✔ central tendency;
- ✔ strict rating;
- ✔ lenient rating;
- ✔ latest behavior;
- ✔ performance dimension order;
- ✔ initial impression;
- ✔ spillover;
- ✔ status effect;
- ✔ same as me;
- ✔ different from me;
- ✔ stigma; and
- ✔ future use.

SUPERVISOR'S CHECKLIST

A checklist will help guide the supervisor in preparing, conducting and following through on performance interviews. (See Figure 9.4)[1]

The checklist covers the stages of:

- preparing for the interview;
- conducting the interview;
- closing the interview; and
- following up after the interview.

Figure 9.4

Performance interview checklist

Preparing for the interview

- ❑ Review the performance plan; e.g., job responsibilities, goals, standards and other performance factors;
- ❑ Review the critical incidents/significant occurrences file;
- ❑ Check these observations to ensure they are free from bias, memory "loss," trait/personality judgments;
- ❑ Review the employee's skills, work experience, training;
- ❑ Consider the employee's performance strengths and improvement areas;
- ❑ Identify the critical points to communicate in the interview;
- ❑ Make notes of developmental ideas;
- ❑ Identify preliminary goals and standards for the next evaluation period;
- ❑ Agree with the employee on a mutually-convenient time for the interview;
- ❑ Provide the employee with a self-assessment tool to prepare for the interview;
- ❑ Review preliminary thoughts about the employee with your manager and ask for guidance and feedback;
- ❑ Ensure there is enough uninterrupted time in your schedule for an unhurried, complete interview; and
- ❑ Arrange to meet in the office, in a private setting.

(continued on page 175)

Figure 9.4 continued from page 174

Conducting the interview

- ❑ Begin the discussion in a friendly way by starting with some small talk, and then noting the session's review/planning purpose;
- ❑ Have the employee "take the floor first" by sharing the self-assessment;
- ❑ Add comments on job performance, accomplishments, employee strengths, improvement areas;
- ❑ Emphasize any areas of major performance concern;
- ❑ Cite specific observations about these areas;
- ❑ Encourage the employee to ask for and give specific feedback;
- ❑ Use open, reflective and directive questions to promote thorough discussion;
- ❑ Discuss any discrepancies between the employee's assessment and your assessment;
- ❑ Ask the employee to identify any support/resource needs;
- ❑ Encourage the employee to discuss personal development goals before suggesting any of your own;
- ❑ Agree on a development/improvement plan;
- ❑ Work together to develop performance goals for the next evaluation period;
- ❑ Give appropriate career advice, without making any promises; and
- ❑ Decide on the final ratings and indicate them on the form;

Closing the interview

- ❑ Make notes during the interview about followup assignments;
- ❑ Ask the employee to summarize what has been discussed and clarify any misunderstandings;
- ❑ Ask if there are any other questions or comments; e.g., often an employee's hidden agenda may not be disclosed unless there are several sincere invitations to "say what's on your mind";
- ❑ Explain how the performance information will be used for compensation and other personnel decisions;
- ❑ Set times for performance progress reports for the next evaluation period; and
- ❑ Conclude on a positive, friendly note;

Following up after the interview

- ❑ Make sure the performance evaluation information for the prior period is complete;
- ❑ Ensure that the performance plan for the next period is complete;

(continued on page 176)

Figure 9.4 continued from page 175

- ❑ Review results with your manager;
- ❑ Sign the form(s) and make copies for the employee to sign, returning one and keeping the other for his/her own file. The employee has the right to notify you if the final copies are not in line with his/her understanding. The employee also has the right to disagree with the final evaluation. His/her signature on the form simply acknowledges that he/she has had an opportunity to discuss it. If the employee refuses to sign the form, ask another person to serve as a witness of the fact that the employee has seen the form but will not sign it. This procedure provides the documentation that may be needed to prove the performance interview did occur;
- ❑ Give copies to the human resource specialist to put in the employee's personnel file;
- ❑ Follow up on any commitments; e.g., training, resources, coaching; and
- ❑ Evaluate your own performance; e.g., preparing for and conducting the interview, and identify areas for improvement.

The last steps of the interview process concentrate on analyzing the entire experience. This is very meaningful in that it helps the supervisor consolidate the learning he or she has gained about performance management. This understanding provides the necessary foundation for getting the next performance period off to a good start for both performance partners.

Note that there is no discussion of salary during this interview other than a comment about the use of performance information for compensation administration. As discussed more thoroughly in Chapter Ten, mixing discussions of performance with salary reviews dilutes the focus on performance.

Problem-solving emphasis

The checklist emphasizes the use of problem-solving in the interview for several reasons. Research about the cause and effect relationships of interview approaches indicates that the problem-solving approach is far more effective than either the "tell and sell" method or the "tell and listen" approach.[2]

In the "tell and sell" method, the interviewer is a judge whose intent is to communicate the evaluation and to get the employee to change. The method assumes that a supervisor is fully qualified to evaluate an employee. Reactions can range from polite acceptance to covert defensive behavior and hostility. If the employee respects the supervisor, the interview has some chance of success. The risks, however, are a decrease in loyalty, independent judgment and mature participation. This method perpetuates existing practices and values.

In the "tell and listen" method, the interviewer also is a judge; however, the intent of the session is not only to communicate the evaluation, but also to encourage discussion. This approach assumes that people will change if there is general discussion. Reactions can range from appreciation for the opportunity to participate to overt defensive behaviors and hostility. The major risk is that the employee may not agree about the need to change. This method does permit the supervisor to change views in light of the employee's responses and does allow some upward communication.

> "The things we stress with supervisors in terms of their interviews with employees are: (1) be straightforward; (2) be honest; (3) help the person maintain his/her self-esteem. Don't ignore things that went wrong — employees must be accountable — but discuss them in a way that a person can still feel OK about themselves; and (4) deal with behaviors, not the individual as a person."
>
> *(MGMA member, small clinic)*

In the problem-solving approach, the interviewer is a helper whose intent is to stimulate growth and development in the employee. The method assumes that discussion of job problems leads to improved performance. Both individuals should react to this approach by using problem-solving behavior. The risks: The employee may lack ideas, or his or her idea of change may be other than what the supervisor had in mind. However, this method helps both individuals to learn since experience and views are shared. Thus, the probability of change is enhanced.

Recall that the classic problem-solving steps are:

- Identify and discuss the problem;
- Encourage the employee to develop possible solutions;
- Agree on one and jointly develop an action plan; and
- Evaluate results and continue if successful, or try another alternative if unsuccessful.

Both the supervisor and individual gain new information and insights as they analyze, brainstorm and decide together. The result has greater potential for success since "two heads are better than one," and since the employee has the opportunity to "buy into" the decision through participation.

This approach, of course, is used throughout the year as the employee and supervisor encounter problems. As noted before, it is especially useful for dealing with major performance problems. It is also the preferred method for discussion of improvement areas during the annual performance review.

Interviewing skills

As discussed previously, listening is a key part of problem-solving. Unless the supervisor asks, listens — and hears — what the employee has to offer in terms of problems and solutions, there will be no mutually satisfactory result.

The supervisor should also listen for feelings and emotions. These might range from the employee's eagerness to hear about a job well done to fear of being scolded about a mistake. The supervisor should listen and respond to these emotions.

If the supervisor tries to understand how the employee thinks and feels about certain issues, there is less likelihood of the supervisor becoming judgmental and creating a defensive climate. Also careful listening gives the supervisor an understanding of an employee's level of self-esteem and his or her need for support.

There are three kinds of questions that facilitate evaluation discussions and give the supervisor the opportunity to listen. They are (See Figure 9.5):[3]

- **Open questions**. These are questions that cannot be answered with a yes or no. The response must be an opinion or expression of feelings. Examples: "What is your opinion of ...?" "How do you feel about ...?" "What do you think caused ...?" "How do you think this could be done differently next time?" These questions allow the supervisor to:
    - demonstrate interest in the employee's point of view;
    - confirm his or her respect for the employee's ideas and feelings;

Figure 9.5

Performance interview questions

Supervisors should use three kinds of questions during performance interviews to facilitate communication:

❶ Open questions.

❷ Reflective questions.

❸ Directive questions.

- stimulate thought about specific issues;
- gain understanding about the employee's needs; and
- encourage a dialog rather than a monologue.

- **Reflective questions**. These repeat a statement the employee has made, but in the form of a question that focuses on the most significant idea or feeling. Example: The employee says, "It would have been better if we had done it differently." The supervisor says, "You're convinced the results can be improved if we modify the procedure?" These questions allow the supervisor to:
  - avoid arguments by responding without accepting or rejecting what the employee has said;
  - confirm understanding of what was said. If the reflection is incorrect, the employee has an opportunity to correct it;
  - encourage clarification or expansion of what was said; and
  - create a dialog that facilitates agreement.

- **Directive questions**. These solicit information about a particular point or issue. They are usually saved until after the employee has finished talking about the subject. Then they can be used to keep communication going, or to obtain specific information or ideas. Example: "If you are convinced the results will be improved, what steps would you take and when would you take them?" These questions allow the supervisor to:
  - get pertinent information about critical areas;
  - challenge the employee to explore ideas, defend statements and contribute suggestions; and
  - illuminate specific facts about an issue.

Open, reflective and directive questions are all useful techniques to draw the employee into a thorough discussion of job performance and personal development.

The supervisor should monitor the amount of listening that's done in the performance interview. Remember the 50 percent rule. The tendency is to listen as a superior, as a judge, to gather ammunition for a winning response. In this case real listening is minimal because the intent is not true communication, but rather to win a battle.

Since the supervisor has asked the employee to do self-appraisal and to come prepared to discuss his or her thoughts, the employee has every right to expect there will be an open discussion and an opportunity to be heard. Employees are much more satisfied with the evaluation process when they participate fully and have an equal chance to discuss what's important to them.

> “It's all in how you say it, when giving feedback. When you smile and say it in a pleasant way, even negative feedback is more acceptable. We suggest that supervisors sit in a way that they have direct eye contact with the employee — not standing up, or across a desk. Then you can discuss performance, not issue mandates. It's a matter of delivery.”
>
> *(MGMA member, medium-sized clinic)*

Training in the needed listening skills can help assure that supervisors can successfully involve employees in discussions. Such training should also cover nonverbal skills. These include:

Body language

Many features of the body — posture, gestures, facial expressions and eye contact — often speak louder than words. Research has shown that people believe what they see (behavior) more than what they hear.

Examples: Leaning forward clues the employee that the supervisor is interested in listening. Direct eye contact provides assurance that the supervisor is giving the employee full attention.

In addition to being sensitive about their own body language, supervisors also must be in tune with the behavior of employees during the interview. They should look for signs of tension, misunderstanding, puzzlement, disagreement. They may need to clarify the body clues.

Example: “You say you agree, but the look on your face and the tone of your voice makes me feel you are not really sure.”

Figure 9.6

Performance interview focal points

This checklist will help the supervisor stay on target during the performance interview:

✓ Am I developing rapport?

✓ Am I concentrating on performance topics?

✓ Am I using facts not opinions?

✓ Am I giving feedback in a nonthreatening way?

✓ Am I encouraging the employee to take responsibility for his/her own behavior?

✓ Am I accepting responsibility for my own behavior?

✓ Am I concentrating on one point at a time?

✓ Am I providing useful information?

✓ Am I encouraging self-assessment?

✓ Am I remembering that my primary role is as performance coach?

Paralanguage

This includes a range of vocal characteristics, including the inflection of words and the tone of voice. These nonverbals can communicate the sincerity of the message conveyed (how something is said is more meaningful that what is said).

Example: The same statement, "I'm so pleased you are here on time," could be said in a way that expresses appreciation — or sarcasm.

Space language

The use of space has special meaning to each culture. In the United States, people prefer to keep some distance between them. However, too much separation is isolating.

Example: If a supervisor sits behind a big desk across from the employee, there is a sense of separation and status rather than partnership. Sitting in chairs facing each other or at a round table provides the best setting for discussion.

Touching

The American culture is not comfortable with touching, particularly in business situations and especially between businessmen and women. Although the connotations may be too sensitive, it is best to use common sense and not use touching as a communication technique, with some exceptions.

Example: Shaking hands at the beginning and ending of the discussion is a useful gesture of friendship and agreement. A hug or a pat on the back as a sign of support or celebration may be appropriate for certain occasions.

Focal points

When conducting an interview, the supervisor should use a mental checklist to stay targeted on key points. These include (See Figure 9.6):

- establish and maintain rapport;
- focus on workplace topics, not personality;

- use facts, not opinions;
- provide feedback in a nonthreatening manner;
- refuse to accept responsibility for the employee's behavior;
- accept responsibility for own behavior;
- keep to one point, one subject at a time;
- provide useful information in understandable amounts at appropriate times;
- promote self-review, self-assessment, self-management, self-responsibility; and
- remember that a supervisor's role is that of resource and coach with improved performance/productivity as the success target.

If the supervisor focuses on these major points, the performance interview should be satisfactory for both individuals.

Summing up

Supervisors who are successful in performance interviewing demonstrate these skills: listening with openness, relinquishing control, proceeding with caution, focusing on observations, using specific examples, encouraging communication, using questions not statements, avoiding arguments, checking for understanding, confronting performance deficiencies — and accepting the challenge to improve the performance of their employees and their own effectiveness as supervisors.

Footnotes

[1]*Robert Maddux.* Effective Performance Appraisals. *Los Altos, Calif.: Crisp Publications, 1986.*

[2]*Marshall Sashkin.* A Manager's Guide to Performance Management. *New York: American Management Association, 1986.*

[3]*Patricia King.* Performance Planning & Appraisal. *New York: McGraw-Hill, 1989.*

Recognition, rewards and recycling

Chapter Ten

Recently a medical practice adopted a CQI approach, and as a result, no longer gave performance ratings that linked to salary increases. Instead, supervisors meet with employees once a year for developmental discussions. Salaries are adjusted across the board annually to reflect competitive wage data, which includes cost-of-living increases. Also, all employees share equally if the gain-sharing plan pays off. There are no raises given to specific individuals. However, there is an incentive program for those who wish to take on extra assignments. There are also rewards for creative innovations. And superior employees are given increased responsibilities, new challenges and the chance to advance as fast as possible. To date, employee performance and organizational productivity are at an all-time high.

The performance of employees is inherently tied to reward. It's a basic human need to know "what's in it for me?" That's healthy self-interest. Individuals have only so much time, talent and energy. They want to use it productively and profitably to take care of a variety of their needs — from survival to self-actualization. Today, there are many reward options to meet these needs.

It is only fair for a medical practice to communicate its understanding of the performance-reward cycle to employees at specific times and ways, including:

- when they join the organization;
- in the employee handbook; and
- at the beginning and end of a performance period.

This communication ensures that there is no misunderstanding about the "performance contract" between the organization and the individual. It should be clear that when the employee helps the organization accomplish its goals, the organization will compensate the employee in a variety of ways. Then, the employee will perform in the desired way again.

Figure 10.1

Current compensation issues

Some of the factors medical practices have to consider today when developing reward systems, include:

- ➞ quality management;
- ➞ performance incentives;
- ➞ pay-for-performance;
- ➞ star performance compensation;
- ➞ recruiting;
- ➞ achievement-support agreements;
- ➞ fixed vs. earned pay;
- ➞ patient service;
- ➞ pay-for-knowledge;
- ➞ compensation package;
- ➞ true merit pay; and
- ➞ retention.

Current issues

These days, the traditional ways of linking performance and reward are changing. (See Figure 10.1) Some of today's issues include:[1]

- How do you measure and reward performance in a transformed work place where quality management cuts across departmental lines, when customers are the most knowledgeable about an individual's performance, when work is no longer seen as a product of individual efforts but as a team effort?
- How do you use incentives for executives, supervisors and workers rather than just relying on standard salary systems?
- How do you design pay-for-performance systems based on factors that lead to group success?
- How do you deal with star performers who are excellent Lone-Ranger performers but may be destructive to team performance?

- How do you use compensation as a strategic tool not only to attract and retain skilled employees but also to ensure that those skilled workers are rewarded for achieving goals that make the group practice succeed?

- How do you help supervisors build achievement-support agreements with employees, agreements based on bottom-line realities of what the assignment is and what "excellent" performance is?

- How do you reduce the amount of guaranteed base salary and increase the amount of "earned" incentive compensation, especially for health care employees such as nurses?

- How do you move to a three-tier reward system based on performance standards that compensate on the basis of achieving organizational goals, team goals and individual goals?

- How do you ensure that key employee behaviors are rewarded such as giving "legendary" patient service that earns life-long trust?

- How do you pay for knowledge when you encourage employees to improve skills and thus organizational productivity?

- How do you build a compensation package with an appropriate ratio of salaries and benefits that works for both the organization and employees?

- How do you move away from traditional methods of paying for seniority/tenure to true "merit pay"?

- How do you retain long-term employees?

Each of these issues poses major strategic questions for medical practice administrators. The decisions may drastically change an organization's performance-reward philosophy, policies and procedures. Basic rule of thumb: Strategically identify how successful performance can best be achieved in the group practice today (e.g., total quality management) and then redesign the performance-reward system to fit the strategy.

Performance evaluations vs. salary reviews

Before discussing these issues in more depth, it is useful to deal with the relationship between performance evaluation and salary evaluation. Historically, performance reviews have been associated with salary reviews. The common practice is to use the performance appraisal review/form as the impetus for determining salary increases.

This approach erodes the contemporary premise of performance management, which is to focus on human resource development. When the review ends with a rating that translates into a monetary adjustment, the attention of the employee is on money not on discussing performance achievements, personal/professional development and new goals.[2]

Supervisors also become so intent on figuring out how to tell employees that their increase is not as high as they expect because of budgets and profitability, that they neglect to put proper emphasis on the performance discussion. This is especially true in these days when salary increases are much lower than in the past, and in some cases, are nonexistent. Some organizations occasionally have to freeze wages and/or even cut wages.

This concentration on salary increases can foster abuses of the system. For example, a supervisor may rate all subordinates as average to superior to avoid having to confront employees with a more accurate evaluation of below average or lower. Or in the case of less availability of funds for salary increases, supervisors may be embarrassed to face employees who have performed successfully but are only receiving token raises.

When salary reviews are on the agenda, employees can focus on little else. All the way through the performance discussion, they will be thinking, "How much do I get?"

Performance interviews, as noted before, should be structured to be positive discussions for the employee and the supervisor. When the subject of salary is the featured attraction, the performance interview will be perceived as anxiety-provoking.

> “As part of our move to CQI, we eliminated merit pay. Instead we have a standard increase. However, it is not automatic. If someone is not meeting standards, they won't get the increase. Not everyone thinks it is wonderful to eliminate merit pay. The big concern for managers is how to handle the outstanding/superior performer. The big concern of employees is about those who don't work as hard.”
>
> *(MGMA member, large clinic)*

Performance data should be used for salary determination, but in appropriate ways and at appropriate times. Performance evaluation for the sake of salary increases should be a distant secondary goal of performance reviews. Performance evaluation is a developmental tool that identifies an individual's past achievements, assesses present strengths, pinpoints areas needing further development and focuses on future goals.

A performance interview should not be a pat on the back and a statement, such as, “You're doing a fine job; keep up the good work. You'll be getting a salary increase of 5 percent effective Monday.”

As discussed in prior chapters, “fine job, good work” have little meaning if there were no specific performance goals and no verification of accomplishment. Success must be specifically defined. The old maxim, “Reward the behavior you want repeated,” is based on letting the employee know which behaviors are expected. It takes time to link the message of performance to reward. Unfortunately, most performance interviews take less than 20 minutes. They should last 40-60 minutes.

Another reason for not doing salary reviews at the same time as performance interviews is budgetary. As part of its strategic planning and budgeting processes, a medical practice will want to look at:

- its ability to pay;
- its competition for employees and competitive compensation rates in the marketplace;
- its strategic plan for generating new kinds of business; and
- its human resource plans for adding new skills/employees, reducing staff, moving to team compensation, etc.

In other words, the concept of performance-reward must be considered at least annually in terms of the big picture. This typically is done a few months before the beginning of a new fiscal year. Once specific goals are identified in the annual strategic plan, the compensation plan can be developed.

It is at this time that the compensation analyst does a market survey to determine what competitors are doing in terms of salaries and benefits and correlates these with updated job descriptions and job evaluations. The result: a revised salary schedule and an updated benefits package. It is also at this time that any major changes are announced to staff; for example, a switch to a pay-for-performance system, a new incentive system, a team-pay system.

Supervisors are then given training related to the year's game plan with the focus on productivity goals expected and the related reward system. These are also communicated to all staff so they understand "how the game is being played now."

During the year as employees' anniversary dates occur, performance interviews are scheduled — to discuss performance. Performance ratings are given; such as, unacceptable, meets standard, above standard, exceeds standard. However, no discussion of salary occurs.

At the time indicated by the budget cycle (often at fiscal year end when the profit margin is known), salary decisions are made by supervisors in consultation with their managers. These decisions are based on the parameters specified by the budget officer. ("We have an average of 5 percent to distribute this year.")

Supervisors and managers review the performance of all employees in a department and make individual judgments on each one. There should not be an effort to force a "bell curve" to fit the budget. Rather each person should be rewarded on the basis of performance. Giving an "across the board" raise means everyone is "average," and that is neither true nor fair — and employees know that. Why should anyone try to exceed expectations if rewards are always average?

All employees then are informed about salary decisions by their supervisors. It is appropriate to do so with a statement related to performance. "We are pleased we are able to reward your superior performance with an 8 percent raise. We really appreciate the effort you make toward achieving the goals we agreed on, particularly in terms of customer service."

If the medical practice presently uses the traditional system of combining performance and salary reviews, it is recommended that supervisors schedule a separate meeting for the monetary discussion within a day or two after the performance interview. This will help to avoid the anxiety attacks and to put the proper focus on performance during the performance interview.

Rewards in a transformed workplace

Because of radical changes in technology and in patient expectations, the work place has been transformed into more lateral and less hierarchical organizations. Decisions that used to be made in the "head office" are now routinely made by the workers who deal directly with customers and who are coming up with new ways to handle business functions; e.g., medical records, supplies, data processing.

In addition, there is recognition that separating out individual contributions to productivity makes less sense since it is the total "service package" that a customer, the patient, buys — it's a team buy. The "buy" begins when the appointment scheduler answers the phone with a smile and arranges for the most convenient time for the patient to come in. It continues when the receptionist makes sure the patient is called by name, is assured the physician, lab, etc., will see her within a few minutes, and is provided with coffee and recent magazines in a "living room" waiting area and not overwhelmed with paperwork.

It continues with the medical staff seeing the patient on time, and taking the time to answer questions, to probe for feelings and concerns and to make the patient feel like she is getting personal attention. It continues with proper processing of bills and records, with followup on findings, with ongoing communication with newsletters, customer satisfaction surveys and reminders of checkups.

This requires teamwork. If one person along the line does not perform effectively and dissatisfies the customer, the organization has failed. Medical practices cannot afford this possibility. Since work is no longer the product of individual efforts, providing only individual rewards is no longer appropriate. Result: team incentives and performance rewards for teams take on much larger significance.

A recently completed survey by the Consortium for Alternative Reward Strategies Research, which studies organizational performance reward plans for nonmanagement employees, found that the trend in compensation planning is to develop performance reward plans that move the organizational unit to improve performance. Historically, people have been perceived as a cost center. They are now perceived as assets, and the change is profound. Organizational performance reward systems are now being seen as a proactive way to stimulate workers to make significant contributions to the organization.[3]

The key: Measuring and rewarding the right elements. Some performance reward experts recommend that each measure should be linked to actions that directly affect a specific customer. For example, a measure of return on assets would be tied to stockholder satisfaction. Service measures would be attached to patient satisfaction. Quality assurance measures would be linked to clinical outcomes. Job-enrichment measures would be tied to employee satisfaction.

Financial measures alone are not adequate. They must be balanced by customer measures. For example, the physician-owners of a clinic may be very satisfied with their return on investment, but their patients may be unsatisfied with patient relations practices.

The consortium study suggests three categories of measurement: financial results, organizational satisfaction and planned operational outcomes such as business performance, teamwork and improvements in the workforce.

Financial measures indicate if the measurement-reward plan is working. However, since employees do not have control over some financial measures and thus cannot influence their rewards, operational measures that they can influence are important.

INCENTIVE PAY

An incentive is defined by Webster as, "something that incites or has a tendency to incite to determination or action." It provides a motive for a person to act. In terms of performance rewards, it should be noted that many incentives are not financial but rather cashless compensation, such as recognition and job enrichment.[4]

Financial incentives are typically (See Figure 10.2):

- variable in amount;
- based on measurable outcomes;
- intended to recognize outstanding behavior;
- promoted in advance; and
- awarded in a lump sum.

Objectives of incentive plans include (See Figure 10.3):

- providing opportunities for additional compensation that will help attract and retain employees;
- motivating participants to achieve specified results;
- improving productivity;
- providing tangible feedback on performance;
- converting otherwise fixed costs (salary) to variable costs;
- encouraging employee involvement;
- managing turnover so that best performers stay and worst performers leave; and
- recognizing outstanding performance.

From an employer's viewpoint, incentives:

- increase productivity/efficiency;
- motivate desired behaviors;
- direct efforts; and
- create variable cost.

Figure 10.2

Incentive pay

Medical practices considering incentive pay should keep in mind that incentives focus on:

- ➡ variable amounts;
- ➡ measurable outcomes;
- ➡ outstanding performance;
- ➡ advance "advertising"; and
- ➡ lump-sum awards.

Figure 10.3

Incentive plan objectives

Medical practices must decide what they want to achieve by having an incentive plan. Objectives can include:

- ➡ recruitment/ retention;
- ➡ motivation;
- ➡ productivity;
- ➡ tangible feedback;
- ➡ variable costs;
- ➡ employee involvement;
- ➡ turnover; and
- ➡ outstanding performance.

> “We may decide to reserve a small percentage of the salary increase budget for special rewards for the 'stars.' Whether you have merit pay or not, you still have to give stars challenges, opportunities for advancement, enrichment, and so forth. Money is never enough as a motivator.”
>
> *(MGMA member, medium-sized clinic)*

From the employee's viewpoint, incentives:

- add discretionary income;
- create real earning potential; and
- keep score.

The key difference between a bonus and an incentive is that a bonus is typically given after the fact based on some general criterion such as "a good year." In contrast, an incentive sets a target ahead of time and the reward is given if the goal is achieved.

Incentive plans for health care executives have been around for some time. For example, a recent survey of 300 hospitals indicated that 39 percent provide bonus/incentive pay to their top managers. These range from 18 percent to 30 percent of salary. Management incentives can be discretionary (whatever the board decides), or formula plans or performance target plans.[5]

Medical practices that have established marketing/sales programs often use classic sales incentives, such as commission plans or goal-attainment plans.

Incentives for all levels of employees are becoming prevalent. Some are well-known, traditional approaches such as profit-sharing plans (distribution of a share of the profits), and gain-sharing plans (distribution of a share of a gain such as labor savings, value added). There also may be other long-term incentive plans such as employee stock plans. Profit-sharing is perceived as less of an incentive since there is usually little direct tie to individual performance. Gain-sharing, in which employees help to set specific goals, is considered to have higher motivational value.

Newer approaches include small group/team incentives and exceptional performance award plans.

Individually oriented reward plans include merit increases, individual incentive plans, pay for knowledge and skill-based pay. Each medical practice should review the various options and determine which ones will work best in their situation. One frequent solution is to provide a combination of all three; e.g., organizational, team and individual rewards.

As medical practices increasingly organize around specific tasks and rely on interdisciplinary teams, the perspective of one supervisor evaluating employees becomes counterproductive. Team goals and team rewards then must become very specific so success is clear to any observer. If conventional incentive programs are used, they just reinforce the employee to try to please the boss, rather than on pleasing the customer.

Combination rewards

Many organizations are experimenting with combinations of individual merit-pay systems and teamwork systems as well as variable and fixed pay, rating and nonrating systems, gain-sharing and individual incentive awards, profit-sharing and employee stock options. Again, the most important factor is what is measured and rewarded.

"Merit" pay in the traditional sense is perceived as less than effective in promoting productivity because of its reputation as "expected or entitlement" pay. Unfortunately, organizations in the past have given merit raises automatically without regard to performance measures. Usually these had nothing to do with meritorious performance, but instead reflected seniority. Length of service was recognized and rewarded. Today few medical practices can guarantee a job for any length of time — and certainly not for poor performers.[6]

A base-pay (fixed pay) system can be used effectively to measure and reward behavioral competency; i.e., the performance factors such as ability to communicate, customer focus, dealing with change, interpersonal skills, ability to work on a team and professional and technical knowledge. These can be linked directly to individual performance and can be used to determine fixed or guaranteed pay.

Such factors for health care professionals might include: quality of patient care as determined by outcomes of quality assurance and utilization review, interdisciplinary communications and case management.

A pay-at-risk reward system is successfully used when tied to accomplishment factors; i.e., specific performance objectives. Such a variable pay approach can be used both as an individual reward system and as a team reward system. For a health care professional, such factors as productivity (number of cases/patients served) and paperwork (number of deficiencies) can be specific performance objectives.

There is a growing trend to decrease the amount of fixed pay and to increase the amount of at-risk pay. A combination plan that reinforces and rewards expected general competencies as well as provides incentives for specific goals covers two important motivational bases for employees. One: The fixed portion takes care of survival and security — the hygiene needs. Two: The variable portion provides the challenge for growth and development that is a true motivator.

Incentives for team performance are goal-based, and thus, provide the motivation to work together effectively to achieve a specific target. Recognizing not only that no one person could accomplish the result, but that rewards only occur if the team succeeds, fosters effective teamwork.

Star and exceptional performers

A challenge remaining for performance reward specialists is how to effectively reward the star performer and the exceptional performer now that the focus has switched to the team rather than the individual. A "star performer" is defined as the traditional Lone-Ranger type who accomplishes a great deal by himself or herself, is uncomfortable working with a team and is often destructive to teamwork.

In the past, this kind of performer (also often known as the "John Wayne" type) was highly valued. Today it is rarely the preferred model of behavior. The problem: This type of behavior is "win for one" rather than for all. However, turning this American competitive ethic into more of a Japanese cooperative ethic is easier said than done, especially with a group of older workers.

There are two possible approaches. One: start converting the MBO/goal-setting performance plan from an individual plan into a team plan. The "star" is given the opportunity to be placed on a career-development promotion track by accepting prime responsibility and rewards for results through a group. Two: At the same time, reward the star with a distinguished-performance award to acknowledge individual performance. Distinguished performance rewards do not necessarily need to be monetary, nor should they just be reserved for stars.

An excellent use of a bonus is to reward performance that is exceptional, after the fact. In this case, management is acknowledging performance "beyond the call of duty." Example: In an emergency situation, such as the illness of a co-worker, the employee pitches in and does the work of two for several weeks. Another example: The employee comes up with an innovation that saves considerable time and money.

> "Theoretically, performance evaluations are not tied to salary reviews; however, the information is taken into consideration. Because the economy is tough, salary reviews actually are disincentives. We have difficulty giving more than 3 percent to 4 percent across a department, and we give no cost-of-living adjustment.
>
> "We are considering a system based on performance standards; e.g., if a person exceeded the standard, there would be a bonus. This would get away from the constant battle of inflation caused by automatic salary increases. And it would get away from the idea of entitlement ... a raise every year."
>
> *(MGMA member, large clinic)*

The bonus can be in the form of a lump-sum cash payment, which is a one-time extra payment. This is preferred rather than a salary raise for this event, which not only is an inflationary practice but also has less motivational force than one "big hit."

The bonus also can be nonmonetary. Example: Time off, a certificate of accomplishment, public recognition. Or a "gift" can be provided, such as a weekend at a resort.

These bonuses are special to an employee when they are surprises — a random hit. Another psychological maxim is to reward selectively and randomly rather than regularly. Once an employee grows to expect a reward, it no longer is motivating. The random hit concept is also called the Las Vegas approach. Studies show that when employees are surprised when doing something right and receive an unusual, and varying reward, they will keep "coming back" — doing the behavior again in hopes of winning the jackpot.

Physician performance-reward

Most recently, attention in physician performance-reward planning has turned from productivity to efficiency, particularly in terms of cost containment. Other factors such as quality of care and utilization review are also being spotlighted.[7]

A thorough discussion of physician compensation is beyond the scope of this book.

Benefits as rewards

More medical practices have found it worthwhile to look carefully at the ratio of salary to benefits in its compensation package. As the movement toward holding fixed base pay steady, while increasing incentive pay continues to evolve, there also has been a move to offer a more diverse and flexible benefits menu.[8]

This movement mirrors what is happening in all types of organizations. Today's work force is much more knowledgeable about the value of benefits and more selective. Employees appreciate having a "core package" of benefits such as medical and life insurance. They also appreciate a "bank" of personal paid days off (rather than the standard number of sick, vacation and holidays). They like flexible work hours to deal with personal and family chores. They like the opportunity to participate in retirement investment plans.

Employees with families are concerned about family issues ranging from parental leave to child care to elder care. Thus, more and more health care organizations are finding it pays off in recruitment and retention to offer these benefits.

Doing a benefits survey each year to determine employee preferences and competitive offerings is critical for any medical practice. Larger practices may want to conduct a formal survey using a questionnaire device. Smaller practices may want to follow the lead of others, as reported in professional publications. Generic information is also readily available; (for example, the annual U.S. Chamber of Commerce Benefits Survey).

Benefit packages change frequently as new needs and services emerge. Employees quickly become aware of what's available elsewhere and will expect the same from their organization.

The general media consistently provide information on benefits, so employees often are as knowledgeable about these trends as supervisors.

Pay for knowledge and skill

Some organizations are now rewarding employees with higher pay and/or promotions for superior job knowledge and performance. They use job knowledge testing measures to determine how well an employee knows his or her job and six-month performance evaluations measure how well it is applied on the job.

The system is based on objective measures of knowledge and performance as stated in the "Knowledge, Skills and Abilities" section of the job description. The focus on knowledge is to ensure that employees truly understand the job content — what the job is all about.

For health care professionals who must consistently participate in continuing education to maintain their knowledge base about new medications, procedures, etc., a knowledge-based compensation system is often used. For example, professionals are compensated on the basis of their value to the organization in experience and knowledge acquired.

Such a system also can be used for any employee at any level. Job content can be defined, measures developed and job knowledge tests given. Those who score highly and apply the knowledge consistently can increase their pay and improve their chance of winning promotions.

Application of the knowledge in a skillful way is another approach. Skill is defined as the demonstration of knowledge. For many years, skill-based pay has been used successfully to encourage employees to add on new skills. With successful performance of each new skill, their pay is increased. This approach is particularly useful in conjunction with cross-training or multi-skilled teams. As noted before, not only does this method give the medical practice more flexibility in allocating its human resources, but also it stimulates personal development.

Cashless compensation

Although all employees need and want monetary rewards for effective performance, they also all need and want psychic pay. They need to feel good about themselves as performers and they want others, especially management, to:

- recognize their effectiveness; and
- acknowledge that recognition with rewards.

People value appreciation for good work as much, and sometimes more, than they value their wages. Thus, supervisors should be encouraged to use a variety of cashless compensation methods. "Cashless" is defined as literally costing nothing, such as a thank you. It also can mean a minimal cost, such as movie tickets or flowers.

The first thing to remember about appreciation as a performance reward is that is must be regular and ongoing. A plant given to an employee after five years of service is not sufficient as recognition for effective performance. As part of their ongoing feedback, supervisors should be giving frequent doses of immediate, honest praise or encouragement. And when employees go the extra mile, this should be noticed and acknowledged openly.

"Recognition" also means indicating an awareness of the employee's existence. Greeting employees each day, using small talk to share personal experiences, taking notice of events in their lives ... gives employees the feeling that their supervisors do know they exist.

Simple forms of appreciation/recognition include (See Figure 10.4):

- verbal thank yous, identifying a specific successful act of performance;
- written notes of appreciation, specific and immediate;
- copies of these notes to upper management and to the employee's personnel file;
- verbal acknowledgment of the performance in public (at a staff meeting);
- a token gift (a single rose, an apple);

Figure 10.4

Cashless compensation examples

There are many types of noncash compensation. Some examples are:

- ➡ verbal and written thank-yous;
- ➡ sending appreciation notes to the employee's family;
- ➡ token gifts;
- ➡ flextime;
- ➡ telecommuting;
- ➡ special training;
- ➡ new duties/roles;
- ➡ personal control;
- ➡ special awards;
- ➡ recognition certificates; and
- ➡ visibility.

Other methods that group practices can endorse include:

- giving time off on the occasion of special performance (letting someone go home early after a big project is done);
- giving supervisors a small amount of discretionary funds for small rewards (movie tickets);
- allowing telecommuting (working at home);
- giving "professional growth" days to attend continuing education or other developmental occasions;
- providing occasional relief from unpleasant/repetitive duties;
- assigning new duties/roles;
- providing on-site access to training;
- giving time off for volunteer/community service assignments;
- having "casual dress" days;
- allowing more personal control over time;
- giving increased visibility through special assignments;
- providing awards/certificates;
- publicizing performance achievements in organizational publications;
- having upper management personally acknowledge the performance; and
- providing tangible reminders of success (printed t-shirts, coffee cups, calendars, pens).

The array is endless. The premise is simple. Give each performer the type of applause he or she prefers. That might be an afternoon off to go hiking in the mountains, or a pizza party for the team. In any case, such psychic rewards should be a regular part of the supervisor's repertoire. They pay off big!

A recent survey found that there are several popular compensation approaches in the health care industry. (See Figure 10.5)

Several of these methods are particularly appropriate for promoting creativity and innovation.

> **Figure 10.5**
>
> **Special forms of compensation**
>
> Medical practices might consider these forms of compensation to encourage innovation:
>
> - cash bonuses;
> - free time off;
> - sabbaticals;
> - retirement bonuses;
> - college education fund for children;
> - research/innovation funds;
> - joint ventures;
> - stock options;
> - royalties; and
> - money pool.

Communicating the performance-reward link

The success of a performance-based reward system depends to a great extent on how it is communicated. Once again, the medical practice's philosophy about performance management is critical. It is vital that information about the system be shared consistently with all levels of employees so there is a clear understanding about the performance-reward cycle and "how we do it here."

Supervisors should be trained and reinforced to remember that both performance and reward are constant throughout the year — not just at the end of the year. Upper management will need to focus each year on the reward system and to ensure it is in line with current trends and competitive practices. Example: If other medical practices are going to flexible work hours, it is time to consider this method carefully.

Summing up

Individuals want to perform successfully. When performance expectations are achieved, employees have the right to expect fair rewards. Every supervisor and organization will want to reward such key behaviors as: progress on projects, cooperation, learning from failure, exceeding goals, solving problems, trying new methods, saving money through ideas and giving legendary customer service.

Thus, every group practice will benefit from designing and maintaining a reward system that truly stimulates performance.

FOOTNOTES

[1]Robert Permut, M.D. "Physician Compensation." *Group Practice Journal*, American Group Practice Association, March/April 1990.

[2]Loretta D. Foxman, Walter L. Polsky. "Performance Appraisals Are Not Salary Reviews." *Personnel Journal*, October 1988, p. 30.

[3]Linda Thornburg. "How Do You Cut the Cake?" *HR Magazine*, October 1992, p. 66.

[4]*Incentive Compensation: Paying for Results*. Wyatt Company seminar, 1990, p. 3.

[5]"Incentives for Hospital Executives." *HR Magazine*, October 1992, p. 23.

[6]Wyatt, ibid, p. 10.

[7]Permut, ibid.

[8]Permut, ibid.

[9]Courtney Price, Alys Novak. *Health Care Innovation and Venture Trends*. Albany, N.Y. 1992, p. 193.

Questions and answers

Chapter Eleven

Here are 25 of the most frequently asked questions about the performance management process and the answers.

Q. What do I do about long-time employees who have been rated as satisfactory or higher using traditional performance evaluation systems, but now we have more specific, higher expectations and it's clear that the employee is really a marginal performer. How do we help the employee adjust — and hopefully improve?

A. First, be aware that legally you would be at risk for dismissing an employee who has received satisfactory evaluations for some time. It's hard to show that performance has dramatically changed during the past 12 months when for many years the employee has been rated as acceptable.

Second, you need to explain to all employees why the performance management process and job expectations have changed (such as the need for clear, specific, high standards of performance in today's very competitive world).

Third, you should work with each employee to develop a performance plan that leads to improvement. Feedback should be frequent and review should be quarterly. In other words, play fair but firm about new expectations and provide constant coaching so the employee has a true opportunity to perform successfully. If not, the consequences should be made clear as well (for example, if there is no improvement, disciplinary action will be initiated).

Q. I have given one of my employees a "very good" performance rating, but my manager says the performance is "standard." The problem is compounded by the fact that I have already shared the rating with the employee. What do I do?

A. It is your fault for not checking with your manager before sharing with the employee. Your organization's performance management process should include a mandatory "review the evaluation with your manager first" rule. This not only gives the supervisor and manager an opportunity to check their perceptions and for the supervisor to pinpoint any deficiencies he or she sees, but also it gives the supervisor a chance to rehearse before the performance interview. In this case, you should be able to prove the "very good" performance by offering concrete behavioral evidence. If you cannot, or if the two of you can't agree, it is best to let your rating stand. Then start fresh by negotiating new, higher expectations with the employee. The two lessons from this experience: (1) The employee should not be penalized because of your error; and (2) the policy of a mandatory discussion with the manager before the performance interview should be upheld.

Q. What if my medical practice has an outdated system that everyone thinks is a joke? What is the best way to stage the update?

A. The first step is to discuss the need for change at a management meeting. It is essential that you get commitment from the physicians and administrators about if, how and when to improve the system. Then get some help right upfront from human resource specialists in the organization, outside consultants and your own employees. Conduct a survey about the present system and get ideas on how it could be improved.

Find examples of plans developed by other organizations. Put together a task force of supervisors and employees to work with the human resource specialist and/or consultant to draft a new plan. Pilot it in a department or two. Revise accordingly. Provide training and materials about the system to supervisors. Communicate via top management to all employees about the new plan and how it will be implemented. Evaluate the results within a year.

Q. How do I make sure our job descriptions and performance evaluation system meet ADA requirements; i.e., actual performance requirements related to physical demands, etc.?

A. Basically, the new ADA law does not require that job descriptions be revised. However, in light of this legislation, it behooves employers to review all job descriptions to ensure they are current and they do describe necessary job requirements, not assumptions. This exercise involves going through each job description and delineating essential and nonessential functions. Example: Is it essential to stand to do filing? Is it essential to hear to be a nurse? Can reasonable accommodations be made?

In job interviews, the same guidelines must be followed. The application cannot ask for disability information. The interviewer can only describe the job requirements and then ask the applicant if he or she can perform as required. Once a person is hired, a medical examination can be required to confirm the ability of a person to do the job. Performance reviews for existing employees also must be based on actual job requirements. Example: If a patient education specialist develops arthritic knees and can no longer stand to teach, is that a detriment to her performance?

Q. I have taken progressive discipline steps with an employee, which have not been successful, and now plan to terminate him. My manager wants to know what the legal risk is.

A. You can reduce your risk significantly by taking two steps. One: The progressive discipline must be fair in terms of giving the employee a true opportunity to work with the supervisor to identify the problem, come up with a solution and work on improvement. This procedure should be carefully documented and should be signed by both the employee and supervisor. The supervisor's manager and the human resource specialist should be involved in the process, and legal counsel, if appropriate. The organization should bend over backwards to demonstrate its good-faith commitment to helping the employee succeed.

Two: The organization should check to see that the present situation is not a drastic reversal from the past. That is, has the employee received satisfactory reviews for several years? If so, the courts will question the reason for the change. They will wonder why the problem wasn't caught long ago.

There is always some risk when you terminate an employee. You can minimize the risk with appropriate documentation and by giving the employee a chance to improve. For example, if the job expectations have changed, an employee must be given a reasonable amount of time to improve.

Q. Why can't you use "attitude" or other personality characteristics in performance evaluations?

A. The simple response is it's illegal to use any performance measurements that are not quantifiable and/or behavioral characteristics or are not job related. "Attitude" can't be measured and focusing on "personality" leads to bias. To say an employee has a "poor attitude" doesn't provide any measurable clues. Rather, say: "The employee answers patient questions in short, blunt statements. The employee does not greet patients with a smile. The employee does not ask if the patient would like further assistance." That's a clear picture of poor behavior. Performance evaluations should focus on results and on behaviors that directly correlate with performance expectations for a specific job.

Q. I was just promoted to supervisor and now am faced with performance interviews that have already been scheduled with employees I have never worked with. I don't think I should be responsible for doing these interviews.

A. Yes, you are. This situation frequently happens and the present supervisor is responsible. There are several ways to handle the situation and they all involve seeking input from others. This could include information from the former supervisor (if not in person, hopefully in his or her files), from co-workers of the employees, from patients or from other supervisors who have interacted with the employees in the context of the job and observed their behavior. Your manager also should be able to provide input. In some cases, you may be able to conduct joint interviews with the previous supervisor.

Q. We hear a lot about pay for performance and we do believe that pay should be fair in terms of the effort expended. However, we have limited dollars for salary increases this year. In the past we have just divided the available money across the board and because there is not much to spread, the motivational impact is small. What other kinds of incentives can we use?

A. Your situation is not uncommon today. Few organizations provide large wage increases, and some even have implemented a wage freeze or initiated layoffs. Most employees know that the average salary increase these days is in the 3 percent to 5 percent range. They are also aware that the job market is very tight. So one of the strong motivators is simply the fact they still have a job.

Other motivators include: time flexibility (flexible schedules), job enrichment (redesigned jobs to make them more interesting), training (professional and personal development, such as skill-improvement workshops), recognition (awards, personal and public acknowledgment of work well done, small tokens of appreciation — flowers, dinner gift certificate, etc.).

Q. Our clinic schedules salary reviews at the same time as the performance review. What are the pros and cons of this approach?

A. Many organizations prefer to handle both reviews at the same time for a very pragmatic reason — then it's all done. Also employees have been trained to expect salary information at the same time. The cons: If salary information is shared during the performance interview, that's all the employee thinks about. The main message, of "How am I doing?" gets lost in the thought of, "How much am

I getting?" It is preferable to have the performance interview first.

You do need performance information to make salary decisions. You may learn something in the interview that would change a predetermined salary decision. Once you have this information, you can put it in the context of what the organization can afford to pay. Because you have had time to think about it, instead of walking into the interview with a figure already in your head, you can make a more thoughtful decision. It is always appropriate to discuss salary generally with the employee, but it is better to explain that the salary review will occur at another time.

Q. We are moving into Total Quality Management. How does this system impact performance management?

A. TQM gurus, such as Deming, suggest dumping all performance management systems. They see them as rigid and as penalizing collaborative, creative group initiatives. Organizations that have had TQM systems for a while tend to convert to a systemwide performance focus with rewards given to the entire team when results are achieved. These group performance/reward methods are supplemented by personal development plans developed with each employee.

Q. I'm not comfortable giving negative feedback. What can I do?

A. Start practicing by giving positive feedback. Many supervisors simply do not have any experience in giving any kind of feedback, so learning to make complimentary comments is a good first step. Try the "I" method tied to a behavior. Example: "I am very pleased when you greet each patient with a smile and a personal comment. You help to make this a friendly environment." The rule is: Praise the behavior you want repeated. So giving feedback about preferred behaviors will really pay off.

Then, when you must give negative feedback, you will be more comfortable because you have practiced making direct statements. In these cases, again use the "I" technique. Example: "I am distressed when you come in late three days in a row. There is no one here to answer the phone and our clients are not being served." Again, the focus is on the behavior, not the person. Practice these comments. Say them out loud to yourself; try them out on your supervisor. Write yourself a script. Deliver the message when you are calm — and be sure to deliver it in private.

Q. What can I do to get "interview insurance" that will help prevent some common human rater errors such as the halo effect?

A. You can never get total insurance against rating errors, such as seeing an employee as an "angel of a worker" because he or she does one thing very well. Human beings have built-in perceptions that are hard to change. Two steps will help, however. One: When you review the employee's evaluation with your manager before the performance interview, ask him or her to double check for rater errors. You can also ask the human resource specialist to review several of your reviews to check for rater patterns you may not see. Two: Get input from multiple sources so your perceptions are balanced with other information, and always remember to focus on behavioral issues.

Q. How can I separate my feelings about a person from the evaluation?

A. First, of course, you should have a results/behaviorally oriented performance plan/evaluation. Ideally, then feelings will not enter into your decision making. It should be clear from the data you have collected what the rating should be. Second, the performance management planning approach should emphasize the employee's self-responsibility for building the plan, reporting back to you on the plan and analyzing his or her own performance. Focus together on specific targets and accomplishments, and the process will be objective rather than subjective. The more input from the employee the better because then he or she will not only have developed the plan but will "own" it.

Q. What is the best way to get physician input for performance reviews?

A. Physicians have little time and little inclination to process more paper. Therefore, provide them with simple, short lists of behavioral statements that they can check off quickly. Provide space for specific examples. Supplement this information with occasional brief discussions with them about, "How's this employee doing?" "What behaviors could be improved?" etc. In short, it is important to educate physicians generally on the performance management process and specifically on how to focus on behavioral expectations.

Q. Peer review has long been used with professionals. How can it be used with all employees?

A. The trend today is to get performance input from all of an employee's "audiences." This is called "360-degree evaluation." One has a unique opportunity to observe the employee on a day-to-day basis — his or her co-workers. They can be given an opportunity to complete a results/behaviorally oriented checklist and to provide specific examples of performance. This technique is particularly important as an organization moves into self-managing teams and other group efforts.

Q. What about input from patients? How important is it?

A. With today's focus on patient service/satisfaction, it is essential that some types of patient surveys be done regularly. Not only does this demonstrate to patients that you want their feedback, it confirms to employees that you are serious about their performance. However, just doing surveys is not enough. The next step is sharing that information with employees and working together on the areas needing improvement. One way to reinforce the focus on patient satisfaction is to design incentive systems that reward employees who have been recognized for outstanding performance by patients. In all cases, you will want to celebrate such performance so the behavior will be repeated.

Q. A new clinic manager joins the organization and says, "My standards are different. You can expect evaluations for all staff to be lower."

A. If your performance management process is based on results/behaviors, this situation should not occur. If results are clear in the past, they should be clear in the future. The data provides the same kind of information. If your PMP takes a general approach, then the "yardstick" is subject to being used differently by a new manager.

In any case, use the opportunity to work with the manager to study the PMP and ensure it focuses on the current performance requirements and expectations of the organization. If the manager decides to change the standards, he or she should make sure that they are realistic, documented and communicated, and that employees have a reasonable chance to improve accordingly.

Q. Employees tend to dislike being rated as "average" on their performance reviews. How should I deal with this?

A. "Average" doesn't say much. What's average to you may be marginal to me. From that viewpoint it doesn't help you as a supervisor. From the employee's viewpoint, being "average" is a putdown. So if your rating scales use this language, change it. Appropriate substitutes are "meets standards or expectations" (which must be clearly defined) or "fully competent" (with a reference point for what "competent" means). "Proficient" is another appropriate term, with a specific definition.

Q. What is the "best" performance evaluation tool?

A. There is no best tool. There are many types that can be used, depending on the need of your organization and the preferences of the managers. There are three included in this manual. The first is a performance-standard method based on the job description. The second is a criterion-based tool describing a range of specific behaviors. The third is a goal-setting tool that focuses on results. The text explains each in detail and provides samples.

Q. How can a manager encourage self-appraisal, self-management and self-responsibility related to performance?

A. Empowerment is the big buzzword today in management. It reflects the need of management to let go of traditional control methods that no longer work in today's lean-and-mean organizations. More important, it reflects the desire of most of today's workers to control their own destiny. In short, the environment is ripe for performance self-responsibility.

When promoting this focus to employees, be sure to position it as a movement to a performance partnership.

Rather than saying "You are on your own," say: "We are in this together. We can win together." Do the performance planning together, encouraging the employee to take the lead in specifying expectations. Give the employee the responsibility for accomplishing the plan, but also be available as a coach and a resource. Encourage the employee to give you regular updates — and show your appreciation for both good news and bad news. Let the person know you are there to help him/her stay on target, and to succeed.

Q. What do I do when an employee doesn't talk much in the performance interview?

A. Many employees are naturally shy and are not comfortable talking about themselves. Others may be intimidated by the occasion, no matter how comfortable you try to make them. Some may have "hidden agendas" that they are afraid to share. An appropriate way to forestall such unresponsiveness is to have the employee complete a self-appraisal form before the session. This step is always recommended. Then have the employee walk through his or her analysis with you. In short, have him or her take the lead using a personal "script."

Be sure the self-appraisal form includes questions about resources, your supervision and other aspects that could affect performance. It also should contain some personal development questions; e.g., what are your plans?

You may be surprised by the employee's input. You may learn something you did not know. You can avoid making errors in judgments/rating and getting egg on your face if you have the employee share first. This gives you some time to consider if your evaluation is very different and to analyze the reasons for any differences.

Q. What do you do when you get conflicting input about an employee's performance? Example: A supervisor rates a nurse as an outstanding performer, but the physician's input is 100 percent different. Or the supervisor rates the nurse low. Then she complains to the doctor and since she is a favorite employee, the physician complains to the supervisor.

A. We hate to say "we told you so," but if you had a results/behaviorally method that forces an objective response, you wouldn't be in this trouble. In this case, you should meet with the other person(s) who provided input and ask for specific behavior examples that will clarify the information. You also may need to ask the human resource specialist to be an impartial party and interview those involved. The lesson learned should be that everyone should agree on expectations and on the way to measure them so evaluations are consistent in the future.

Q. This employee is my best friend, but her performance has not been so stellar this year. What if I am honest? Do I ruin our friendship?

A. The classic response would be, "A supervisor should not be a friend to an employee." In any workplace, that's difficult to pull off, and particularly in small clinics where there is a "family" atmosphere. An appropriate strategy is to sit down with the employee/friend and say, "I am your friend. But in this conversation, I need to wear my supervisor's hat. And in this role, I need to share with you that I am concerned about your performance. Let's review it and see where the trouble spots are and then discuss how you can work out an improvement plan and how I can support it."

Q. What if I run into an employee who is never satisfied with the evaluation? He always sees his performance as being two notches above where I see it? He may even see himself as perfect.

A. You may occasionally encounter employees who always see their performance as better than you do. Your challenge is to help them be realistic. Let the data lead to discovery. Have the employee "prove" perfection by presenting the evidence. Again, the emphasis is on self-responsibility and on clear expectations. The employee has to satisfy himself first that he hit all the marks. Then you will be more than willing to review the actual results and confirm his "perfection."

Q. What do you do about supervisors who simply never get around to doing performance evaluations because they are "too busy?"

A. This is unacceptable behavior — and dangerous, too. For legal reasons, you need to prove that you are serious about your performance management process. One way you guarantee this is by ensuring that supervisors get their evaluations done on time. The human resource specialist should be responsible for monitoring this effort. If supervisors are not cooperative, their managers should be notified. To reinforce the point, supervisors should be rated on this factor in their performance interviews. Some organizations even dock the supervisor's pay if the evaluation is late.

Additional MGMA resources

Following are additional human resources materials and services available through Medical Group Management Association/Center for Research in Ambulatory Health Care Administration/American College of Medical Group Administrators.

Ambulatory Care Nursing Standards and Performance Evaluations

by Karen Knutson, Judy Steiner, Linda D'Angelo, Marie DesChamps, Sandra Matherly and Jane Rochester.

Published by the Center for Research in Ambulatory Health Care Administration (CRAHCA), this handbook provides administrators and managers with a program for evaluating the performance of nursing service personnel within an ambulatory care setting. The evaluation technique presented utilizes the development of work standards that are measurable and identifiable for each job. This method of appraisal takes into account the changes that occur as an employee's tenure and experience increase. The positions presented range from administrative nurse manager to medical office assistant. The book includes performance standards, job descriptions, evaluation tools and a bibliography. Book, 1987

Educational Programs

Human resource issues are addressed at MGMA's annual conference, section conferences, specialty meetings and the Human Resource Society's annual conference.

The Group Practice Job Description Handbook

by Courtney Price, Ph.D.

A source to help you prevent "reinventing the wheel," this publication gives you over 250 sample job descriptions for over 140 personnel positions in group practice. All levels are covered with both a generic job description and an actual sample form used in a group practice. Information on the how and why of job descriptions is also given. Book, 1991

The Group Practice Personnel Policies Manual

by Courtney Price, Ph.D.

This manual is designed to help group practices develop personnel policy manuals and handbooks that meet the unique needs of a medical group. The chapters contained in the guide explore the current issues and thinking behind sound personnel policies today and explain some of the particular needs facing the health care profession. Compensation, leave and employee and labor relations are just a few of the many topics covered in the guide. Each section includes extensive samples which can be adapted to a group's own needs, or used as they appear. Book, 1991

Human Resources Society of Medical Group Management Association

The Human Resources Society (HRS) was created by Medical Group Management Association in 1981 to give administrators the information needed for human resources management. *The Human Resources Society* offers the administrator legislative updates, networking opportunities and education programs tailored to human resource management.

In-House Supervisory Training Program

The *In-House Supervisory Training Program* is designed to enable the medical group administrator who has no prior hands-on training experience to act as a staff development trainer for supervisors in his or her group. This program is unique because it is specifically developed to train supervisors who work in a medical group setting. The program consists of *The Guide: In-House Supervisory Training Program* by Mary Alice Krill, Ph.D., FACMGA, creator of the program, which provides the trainer with background information about the different sections of the program and specific tips to conducting each module. *The Manual: In-House Supervisory Training Program* is a detailed document that leads the trainer through each step of the training process; the accompanying audio tape helps participants perform their functions, as "actors" or "observers" when the "modules" are played out. Also included are enough training materials to train six supervisors. Training package, 1991

Personnel Postscript

To keep personnel manuals and employee handbooks up-to-standard, *Personnel Postscript* brings you the latest, most current information about personnel issues in medical group practice management. The quarterly newsletter supplements *The Group Practice Personnel Policies Manual.* Newsletter, Quarterly

For more information on:
Publications - 303-397-7888
Educational Programs - 303-397-7881
Human Resource Society - 303-397-7894

or write:

Medical Group Management Association
104 Inverness Terrace East
Englewood, CO 80112-5306

Index

A

B

C

H

I

J

K

L

M

N

O

P

S

T

U V W

About the authors

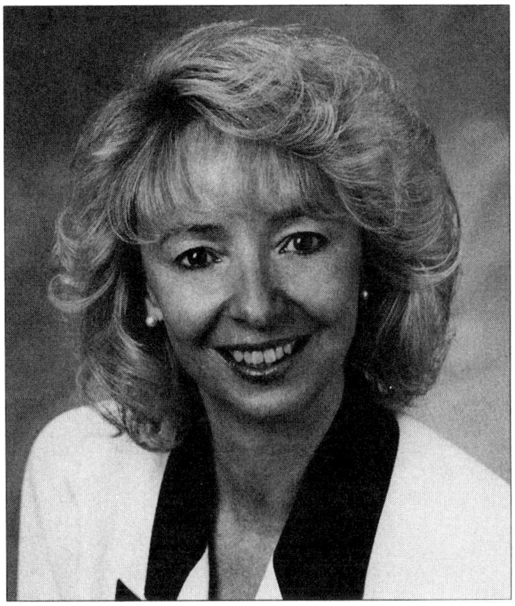

CourtneyPrice, Ph.D., is the Director of the Institute of Entrepreneurship and Creativity and a Professor of Management in the School of Business at Metropolitan State College of Denver. She is an internationally recognized management writer, lecturer, and consultant. She has conducted management seminars on creativity, innovation, productivity, human resource management, and entrepreneurship world wide for corporations, government, and professional organizations.

Dr. Price is a veteran in healthcare management consulting with numerous healthcare providers on productivity, innovation, human resource issues, and implementing entrepreneurial ventures. Her research on innovative trends and new ventures in the healthcare industry was recently featured in *Hospitals Magazine* and *Modern Healthcare.*

Dr. Price has won literary awards from the American Hospital Association for *The Management Guide for Developing Personnel Policies, Procedures and Employee Handbooks.*

She co-authors *Personnel Postscript*, a quarterly healthcare update service for human resource professionals, published by Medical Group Management Association. Dr. Price is also co-author of a software program for writing business plans entitled, *Venture.*

In addition to her books, Dr. Price writes a nationally syndicated weekly column for the *Rocky Mountain News* entitled, "Entrepreneurs Ask."

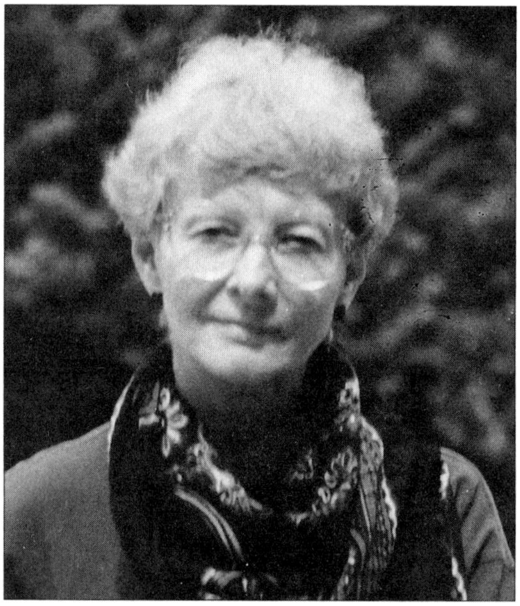

Her collaborator on many of these ventures, who is serving as co-author of this book, is Alys Novak, M.B.A. Her years of experience in business journalism and management consulting have included many assignments in the health care field. Presently she is a Program Manager for the Visiting Nurse Association of Denver and is also an instructor at Metropolitan State College of Denver, specializing in courses such as performance management and compensation administration. She is the co-author, with Price, of the recently published book, *Health Care Innovation and Venture Trends* as well as a co-author of the text, *Nonprofit Financial Management.*